Broken Bodies /
Shattered Minds

A Medical Odyssey
from Vietnam to Afghanistan

Ronald J. Glasser M.D.

Former Major, United States Army Medical Corp

History Publishing Company
Palisades, New York

Published in the United States by
History Publishing Company LLC
Palisades, NY 10964
www.historypublishingco.com

SAN: 850-5942

  Glasser, Ronald J.
    Broken bodies/shattered minds : a medical odyssey
  from Vietnam to Afghanistan / Ronald J. Glasser.
    p. cm.
    Includes bibliographical references and index.
    LCCN 2011927256
    ISBN-13: 9781933909479
    ISBN-10: 1933909471
    ISBN-13: 9781933909486 (e-book)
    ISBN-10: 193390948X (e-book)

    1. Soldiers--Wounds and injuries--United States.
    2. Soldiers--Health and hygiene--United States.
    3. Soldiers--Mental health--United States. 4. United
    States--Armed Forces--Medical care. 5. Vietnam War,
    1961-1975--Health aspects. 6. Afghan War, 2001---Health
    aspects.   I. Title.

      UH215.G53 2011   355.3'45'0973
                        QBI11-600091
  Printed in the United States on acid-free paper

9 8 7 6 5 4 3 2

First Edition

Broken Bodies /
Shattered Minds

*A Medical Odyssey
from Vietnam to Afghanistan*

In admiration and respect for Dr. Michael McCue,
arguably one of the finest neurosurgeons in America,
who cares for the wounded of Iraq and Afghanistan through the
Department of Defense Heroes Program
and who edited these pages for content and accuracy—paragraph by
paragraph and sentence by sentence—with a surgeon's scalpel.

CONTENTS

FOREWORD

In a country that over the last forty years has grown more distant, becoming less involved and less concerned about its military, Dr. Glasser's newest book is both a cautionary tale as well as a powerful redemptive work. Expertly crafted, there are sections of this book that could be used by active duty personnel to teach past military history—both successes and failures—as well as become a primer on current strategy and tactics, including the liturgy of the ever-changing, ever-more-deadly, and ever-more-challenging wounds of war.

The connections with our past wars, particularly between Vietnam and our current wars, are valid on factual grounds. We never had enough troops in Vietnam and we do not have enough troops in Afghanistan. We never sealed the borders in Vietnam and we cannot seal the borders in Afghanistan. We never had a real exit strategy in Vietnam and we clearly do not have an exit strategy of any merit or validity for Afghanistan. We trained a South Vietnamese Army that lasted a year. The Iraqi Army will last a few months, the Afghan Army a few weeks.

Dr. Glasser writes with a quiet elegance, factual precision, and emotional restraint that make this a book of great power and greater substance. It will enlighten, amaze, and trouble you—and it is a book America needs now, more than ever.

—*Lt. General Harold G. Moore, U.S. Army (Retired)*

1.

FORTY YEARS OF WAR

Why write anything? For those who aren't there, it's like it isn't happening, and for those who are, it's like it doesn't count. But there have been 1.9 million soldiers and marines deployed to Afghanistan and Iraq over the last decade, with over 5,000 killed, some 300,000 wounded, another 250,000 diagnosed with PTSD and over 300,000 with traumatic brain or concussive central nervous system injuries, along with amputees approaching levels not seen since our Civil War. These are by any measurement or comparison truly enormous numbers. You'd think that so many wounded, if not dead, would be hard to ignore. But they are.

Yet, these numbers do count, not only to the families of those killed and wounded, but also to the nation. The Iraq and Afghanistan wars have become a 3 trillion dollar war that we can continue to ignore or simply write off. There will be both a moral and economic reckoning before these wars are over and we all finally do go home. And that is what this book is about, that reckoning—the physical, mental, and psychological costs of these wars, those real and those invisible wounds, the anguish and persistent suffering. Unlike all our other wars, the real legacy of Iraq and Afghanistan is not the graveyard but the orthopedics ward, the neurosurgical unit, and the psychiatric outpatient department.

This is a book about forty years of war. It is written from the bottom up rather than from the top down. These are the stories of the soldiers and the marines who actually did and still do make the fight, and those doctors, nurses, and medics who are there when they die and then simply turn around and go on to try to save those who have somehow managed to survive. It is not a book of memoirs or even remembrances, nor is it a book of narrative non-fiction; these stories are no more and no less than the truth. Everything in this book happened. All the numbers and facts are real.

But war is a brutal business. So in places I've changed unit designations in the hopes of protecting those we have once again sent out to the Edge of Empires. In "All the Toms" and "All the Jakes," the real Tom and Jake asked me not to use their names. I interviewed both a number of times. They not only survived their deployments, they survived intact. Tom is now in Special Forces and Jake will soon be leaving the Marines.

Yet, because of the confusion caused by the Army's and Marine's multiple deployments, I merged Tom's and Jake's stories with those battles and firefights they had heard about or those fought by other squads or platoons in their company, regiment, or brigade in order to give a clearer understanding of a history that had so quickly overtaken both the strategists as well as those making the fight. What is unchanging and unchangeable is that those things Tom and Jake saw and experienced were exactly the same things that were seen and experienced by every soldier and marine I talked to or interviewed. There is a terrible democracy to war.

The wounds though, those mangled arms and lost legs, the burns and penetrating head wounds, the transected spinal cords, the grief and the depression, the traumatic brain injuries, the blindness and the pain, all speak for themselves. As for the dead, we still have our poets:

You think their dying is the worst thing that can happen.
Then they stay dead.

2.

The Late Great 1968 / Welcome to the Army

During the decade of the Vietnam War, the Selective Service System swept up some 20,000 draftees every month! Over 4 million troops were sent to Southeast Asia to fight, to die, and be wounded in Vietnam, Laos, and Cambodia. Whatever has been written or said about Vietnam, there was a regular harvesting of young men and little else before it was over.

By the time I was drafted in the summer of 1968—the year that I completed my medical specialty training and ended my military deferment—the Army was not only running down, but running out of virtually everything, including physicians. The chief of the county hospital where I had finished my training as a pediatrician wanted me to stay on at the hospital to care for the pediatric patients of the county's indigent population. He actually sent a letter to the Pentagon, through our Senator, asking for an additional two-year deferment for me.

The next week, he received a certified letter from the Pentagon that said right up front, "Absolutely not ... in case you haven't noticed we have a war going on and every citizen, including every physician, is expected to do his duty." As it turned out, that wasn't quite everybody.

The 101st Airborne, The 82nd, The First Air Cav, The 25th Division, The 9th, The American, and the 173rd Airborne Brigade, because of deferments given for being in school, in the National Guard, having asthma, having a bad back, being flat-footed, almost anything that a family could get a doctor to document, were made up of eighteen- and nineteen-year-old blacks from Cleveland, Detroit, and Cincinnati, Hispanics from East Texas, and poor southern whites. Virtually every Field, Company, and General Grade Officer was from a small town of less than 7,000.

There were few soldiers in Vietnam from families of wealth, power, prestige, or privilege. There was actually a time in early 1969 when the Marines (that had been since their beginnings a volunteer outfit), because of deaths and injuries, were running out of trigger-pullers—and sergeants in induction centers across the country would walk down the line of new draftees and every third one, tap them on the shoulder and say "Marine" … "Marine" … "Marine." At the time, that was pretty close to a death sentence and the draftees knew it. There were some, though, who viewed the military as a stepping-stone to a political career. Again, they were mostly from the South—and there weren't very many of those.

In early 1967, Secretary of Defense Robert McNamara lowered the IQ standards for induction into the military, giving the Army over the next three years an additional 100,000 new draftees each year. They were called "McNamara's One Hundred Thousand." Many of these soldiers couldn't read, and the military had to print comic books with pictures rather then printed copy to get these draftees through basic training.

The least jarring reason for lowering IQs was that the Army simply needed trigger-pullers as cannon fodder; the most cynical was that it allowed the ongoing college deferments to continue, despite the ever-increasing demands for more and more troops on the ground. Three years after the program began, and only after the resignation of McNamara, the low IQ induction program was stopped when it was discovered that these soldiers were killed or wounded at three times the rate of drafted personnel with standard IQs. Even the Army didn't want their troops killed or wounded just because they couldn't quite figure it out or get it right.

But Vietnam was that kind of war—full of all kinds of stupidity, obfuscations, nonsense, suffering, and death. It seemed after a while to be a war that no one could really understand and very few were able to explain. It did seem though that Vietnam went on for so long because it wasn't the kids of those with power and political clout or even the policy makers who were going to 'Nam, but someone else's kids. That kind of thing always makes it easier to start a war, and definitely makes it easier to keep one going even as it begins to fall apart.

I received my orders to report to the Medical Student Detachment at Fort Sam Houston, San Antonio, Texas, for six weeks of basic training on or before August 12, 1968. I had gone home to Chicago to say goodbye to my parents before leaving for the Army. It was right after the brutal clash between the police and the peace-activists at the National Democratic Convention. The anti-war riots had continued not only in Chicago, but across the country. On my way to the airport there were still National Guard units out on the streets who had used their 50-caliber machine guns to shoot out street lamps just the night before.

I had no idea why we were in Vietnam. I think that at the time it had to do with something that had happened in the Gulf of Tonkin—one of our destroyers that had been attacked—or it was the domino theory of stopping the communists before they took over all of Southeast Asia, or maybe it was just to show the Russians that we really meant business. During my two years in the Army I never did figure it out, nor was it ever really explained to me or anyone else, from company commanders to the grunts pulling the triggers. What I was sure of was that it didn't have much to do with the Viet Cong or the North Vietnamese drifting across the Pacific on rafts to attack California.

But I do remember thinking that day driving to the airport, looking out at the military road blocks on State Street, that despite all the pronouncements of military success in winning over the hearts and minds of the South Vietnamese people, that some clearly weren't yet convinced. For better or worse though, the war was finally on everyone's mind. It certainly was on mine.

I took a commercial jet from Chicago to San Antonio, unaware that the stresses of Vietnam were already forcing the military to begin cannibalizing medical units and hospitals across the world to find enough physicians for 'Nam, as well as the hospitals in the Evacuation Chain and the large military hospitals in the States. From the airport in San Antonio, a bus took me and other new medical draftees and soon-to-be officers onto the base at Fort Sam to begin basic training. The song on the radios in Texas was Pete Seeger's "Waist Deep in the Big Muddy and the Big Fool Says to Push On."

I entered the Army six months to the day after the start of the Tet Offensive, when the Viet Cong overran some 125 U.S. bases, occupied the U.S. embassy in Saigon, and took over the northern South Vietnamese city of Hue. It would take months of brutal fighting to retake all the bases, as well as Hue itself. Some 90,000 Viet Cong were killed in the fighting. After the Marines retook Hue, you could stand on the east bank of the Perfume River and look out over the city on the west bank and not see a wall left standing that was over three feet high.

I remember a sergeant in the 101st Airborne who had been shot through the chest telling me that after his unit took back their base camp in the Central Highlands they had put up a sign near the entrance to the rifle range "45 VC Killed down Range … Go Airborne." But he also understood that if the enemy could make it to your rifle range something had gone terribly wrong, no matter what kind of sign you put up.

The Military Command in Saigon called the turning back of the Tet Offensive and the recapturing of the main U.S. bases in the south a "great military victory." But it was not lost on anyone that if the Viet Cong could pull this kind of thing off once, they could certainly pull it off again.

We were clearly paying a very high price for that kind of "success." By the time I left Fort Sam, the number of U.S. troops killed in Vietnam since Tet had doubled. Since the first deaths of three advisors to the South Vietnamese Army in 1959, the total numbers had reached over 25,000.

At Fort Sam, the pressure was put on those of us with permanent duty station orders for bases outside of the Continental United States—but not Vietnam—to either voluntarily extend an extra year, or have our orders changed to 'Nam. Those with orders for stateside medical facilities were to keep their orders and the usual two-year military commitment.

I had orders for the military hospital at Camp Zama, Japan, to serve the children of the dependent military population as well as government and contract Department of Defense personnel. The carrot was that a three-year tour allowed you to bring along your family as military dependents and at government expense. The stick, of course, was getting killed or wounded serving elsewhere.

About half of us who had arrived at Fort Sam already had orders for Vietnam. There were a few specialists, mostly orthopedic and cardiovascular surgeons, but the majority of those with orders for 'Nam were right out of medical school, with an internship in internal medicine or surgery. They were sure to be in a battalion aid station or out in the bush with the troops. In a very real way, they were the expendable ones and everyone knew it.

The Army is not a democracy. If a company commander believed that his troops would perform better if they had a real doc with them rather than medics, then the docs went out with the patrols, getting shot at just like everyone else. What none of us knew at the time was that the combat troops protected their doctors even better than they protected themselves.

From that first day at Fort Sam, you didn't have to ask who had orders for 'Nam. They were the ones who had a real seriousness about them—if not yet a sense of doom, at least a kind of patina of fear. They didn't joke about the unbelievable military nonsense, like the map-reading course that started out with a poster showing a map under the heading, "This is a Map."

Those of us without orders to Vietnam actually stayed away from them, telling ourselves that it was best to leave them alone, but really because we had no idea what to say or what to offer. They were the ones who had clearly lost, even though there was a general rumor going around that only three or four docs had been killed in 'Nam.

The chances of getting killed as a physician were small. But if it was you, it was 100 percent. That much was clear to all of us. But as a surgeon with orders for one of the military hospitals in Germany said, "They don't have to kill you. Did you ever see a one-armed surgeon?"

The seeming randomness of who was going to 'Nam and who was going somewhere else was the first sense we all had that war was at best a crapshoot. Turn right instead of left and you could be hit; linger a bit out on patrol or move too fast and you'd be the one blown up.

What I would soon learn about war and what was to prove so terrifying was not the "fog of war" that the military philosophers and historians talk about, or that no battle plan lasted longer than the firing of the first bullet or the dropping of the first bomb. It was the simple fact that it really didn't matter how clever you were or how talented or even how well-trained or committed you were.

Whether you were killed or wounded remained what it has always been—an exercise of simple luck. Bend over to pick up a dropped cigarette lighter and the bullet that would surely have killed or crippled you cracks harmlessly out over your back. Forget for a moment to look down because you're distracted by a noise or a glint of sunlight off a wet leaf, and no matter how diligent you've been, you'll miss the wire stretched across the track or the detonator plate half buried in the dirt. If you are in the wrong place at the wrong time, you are doomed and there is little you can do about it. It was said that during the Second World War, the marines on their way to Iwo Jima already viewed themselves as dead.

Sheer chance on the battlefield is not only the final arbiter of winning or losing, but also, of living or dying. When Napoleon was asked what quality he admired most in his generals, he answered without hesitation: "luck."

Fort Sam was both an astonishing transition and a personal conversion. You get on the bus as a civilian and you get off the bus as part of the Army. That much was made clear to all of us from the moment we were greeted by sergeants who seemed to understand, even if we didn't, that not only were we all in the Army now, but that it was an army at war.

I remembered during those first few weeks of basic training that in Tolstoy's *War and Peace,* General Kutuzov, having decided that there was no choice but to burn Moscow to save Russia, was smart enough to understand that the decision to burn the capital wasn't made at the moment he realized there was no alternative, but at some other moment when he'd made that wrong decision or the mistake that had led to this desperate act.

Tolstoy was either clever or smart enough to know that it is never the last circumstance that forces your hand, but the previous half-dozen poorly thought-out actions or opportunities missed or ignored. It's these that precede the need to have to act foolishly or desperately.

That was exactly the way I felt as basic training took me and everyone else deeper and deeper into the war. How did I get here? How did we all get here? What had we been thinking and where had we been looking? How had we all so completely missed what should have been so obvious? I was baffled.

I had attended one of the best undergraduate schools in the country and one of the most prestigious medical schools. I had just finished a much-sought-after internship and residency at a world-famous hospital, and had my whole personal and professional life ahead of me.

How did I end up in Texas? How was I suddenly learning about weapons, bullets, fragmentation wounds, crew-served weapons, potable water, and the best way to navigate at night using a flashlight, a compass, and a back azimuth?

It was clear from the long silences during the different lectures and presentations that those going to 'Nam felt that same kind of bewilderment and confusion even more deeply than I did and, quite honestly, all the rest of us. This was not what they, or any of us, had bargained for.

Still, I drew some kind of comfort, if not understanding, from Trotsky's admonition to the youth of Russia and all of Europe at the beginning of World War I: "You might not be interested in war, but war is interested in you." Maybe we all should have paid more attention.

But the truth was that suddenly the war was now everywhere for all of us. It was increasingly in the daily class work and formations, where Vietnam, while not quite the main point of discussion, was certainly the main focus. It was in the lectures and conversations and in the knowing looks of the NCOs and the officers. Med-evac choppers and gunships were constantly flying over our heads, and on occasion, we would see tanks and armored personnel carriers on the roads, as well as artillery batteries set out in the middle of the fields surrounding the base. It was in the crew-served weapons demonstration out on the weapons range, when the instructors set up machine guns and completely obliterated human-shaped targets at 1500 yards, that the reality of what we were now part of suddenly hit all of us. One of the instructors explained that automatic fire was sometimes erratic which might "give you a chance to survive, but that was not a likely outcome, not if the enemy knew what they were doing."

We were shown films of what bullets could do to blocks of gelatin and pigs and sheep. They could have shown us films of the effects of artillery barrages or roadside bombs or even of 120-mm tank rounds, but to those of us who were uninitiated—and that meant all of us—the Army was showing us what would be the classic wounds of fighting in a jungle where those who are shooting at you are looking right at you, or waiting in ambush, or alongside the edge of a trail or path. What we were watching being done to the animals and the blocks of gelatin was what would be happening to those we would be trying to save. To take a round through the chest or abdomen and certainly the head was to be a mortal wound. If you were not killed outright, you would bleed to death, and that happened all the time.

The Army knew enough about Vietnam to know that the VC and NVA would not be using artillery or fighter-bombers, tanks, or helicopter gunships; they would be using light machine guns and AK-47s. The wounds would be from bullets, so the animals being shot and the blocks of gelatin being exploded by the impact of a high-velocity round was the reality of what would be happening to our troops. Small arm and automatic weapon rounds were to be the signature wounds of 'Nam and that meant that you would either be killed right there where you were hit, or you would be dead before the med-evac chopper could get in to take you to the nearest surgical or evac hospital.

Brain injuries of any kind in Vietnam were universally fatal, either because they would be the result of taking a round through the head, or because they were associated with multiple chest or abdominal injuries. It would take forty years and another two wars for traumatic brain injuries to become the signature wound that resulted from sending more of our soldiers and marines out to another "Edge of Empires."

In forty years it would be IEDs, roadside bombs, and suicide bombers. There would be nothing very high-tech anymore and nothing that you couldn't put together in your own kitchen or bathtub or steal from an ammunition dump. All you would really need would be a couple of 155-mm shells along with some home-made high explosives, some wires, maybe a cell phone and a detonator cap. The enemy wouldn't even have to show themselves, and they definitely wouldn't have to be close enough to actually be shooting at you.

What those of us going to 'Nam in the late 1960s and early '70s to care for the wounded—whether as battalion surgeons out in the boonies or at the surgical hospitals or as specialists in the different Evac hospitals along the medical evacuation routes back to the states—would soon find out, was that our soldiers and marines would be shot or wounded by small anti-personnel booby-traps, mortar rounds, or satchel charges thrown or laid by sappers, along with the more than occasional rocket-propelled grenade. The wounded that we saw in the different hospitals would be the ones who did not bleed to death within minutes of being hit. The types of wounds were the reason that throughout the whole of the Vietnam War over 52,000 U.S. soldiers and marines would be killed, while the final tally of overall casualties would be less than 2.4 wounded survivors to every death. The majority of those severely wounded in 'Nam did not survive. They died where and when they were hit. You wouldn't need the new poly-trauma units or the numbers of occupational and physical therapists or the large numbers of orthopedic or neuro-surgeons for Vietnam that you would later need in Iraq and Afghanistan. The graveyard was to be the real legacy of 'Nam.

Entering the Army in the 1960s was like having entered some kind of parallel universe that none of us had noticed, but that had always been there. But the true reality of what we were now so much a part of, as well as what we had clearly become, occurred out on the infiltration course. Live rounds from 30-cal-iber machine guns were cracking through the air less than six feet over our heads. It had been made crystal clear to all of us that, as medical officers, we were not to even try to deal with a combat situation. If under attack, we were to take orders from any trained military personnel, even if that soldier was no more than a private. In combat, we were to listen and obey whatever the private asked and whatever he ordered.

"You have to know how to do this, or you and those around you will be killed," was how simply it was put. What "this" was became clear out on the infiltration course, with those rounds firing over our heads and explosive charges going off in the bun-kers surrounding us as we crawled forward through the dirt and dust of Central Texas. It was noisy and it was scary. We were reminded before we started that these were live rounds being fired over our heads and that whatever happened, we were not to stand up.

It wasn't Anzio or Normandy, but it was just as real. It was not naïve or romantic to say that for most of us, to have death no more than a few feet away was not only unnerving—it was transforming. All you had to do was just stand up and you would be gone. That kind of thing can change not only what you think about, but *how* you think. You get through the barbed wire part of the infiltration course by rolling on your back and wiggling your way forward under the strands of barbed wire, being careful where you put your hands, to stay clear of the sharpened barbs.

Most of us had finished the course, when an overweight obstetrician, forgetting to turn completely onto his back, got caught on the wire and couldn't move forward or backwards. Above the sounds of the machine gun firing and the detonations of explosive charges in the bunkers, we all heard a plaintive, terrified voice, "I'm caught … help me … I'm caught on the wire … I can't move … help me."

For a moment we all froze, not sure that the panic in the voice wouldn't lead to his doing something really stupid. At that moment, I clearly understood that the Army was not in the business of killing obstetricians, any more than it was in the business of killing anyone else other than the enemy. Standing there at the end of the course, sweating and covered with dirt, I was confused and troubled by the realization that they could have stopped the firing a couple of minutes earlier to be able to go safely out on the course to cut him free. But then I realized that the NCOs in charge of the course wanted to make a point with us young smart-alecky docs. And they did.

As it turned out, we were all caught on the wire. During the fourth week of basic, during morning formation, those of us who had arrived at Fort Sam with orders for a two-year tour of duty at hospitals and medical facilities outside of the continental United States were told to remain at attention. Those who had come to Fort Sam with orders for 'Nam or for military facilities within the continental United States were dismissed and allowed to go on to breakfast.

Virtually all of us who remained had graduated from medical school in the mid-1960s and accepted Berry Plan deferments to finish our specialty training before being drafted. We had been convinced that the two or three additional years of deferment that we were signing up for would buy us enough time so that when our deferments ran out, we would have everything we wanted—we would be board-eligible in our chosen specialty and the war in Southeast Asia would surely be over. It seemed a good deal all the way around. As it turned out, we were only half-right.

At the time most of us had applied for the Berry Plan, General Westmoreland, the U.S. Commander in Vietnam, had asked for 100,000 troops to win the war. The next year, it was another 150,000. By the time we reached Fort Sam, he had asked for, and President Johnson had given him, an additional 300,000, taking the total number of military personnel fighting in Vietnam to more than half a million.

There were clearly stresses working their way through a system that had sent 500,000 troops to Southeast Asia. That morning, we were to learn about one of them—specifically, that the Army was running out of physicians to take care of the increasing numbers of casualties, as well as being able to fulfill all their other worldwide obligations.

The major in charge of the Medical Student Battalion stepped to the front of our formation and announced without the slightest hesitation, confusion, or embarrassment that those officers with orders for permanent duty stations other than Vietnam, but outside of the continental United States, would have their orders changed to the 90th Personal Replacement Vietnam. Once in country, those officers would be assigned as needed, unless they agreed voluntarily to extend their tour of active military duty from two to three years. Those of us with such orders were to come to his office by 1600 the next day to personally give him their decision.

That was it—an extra year in the Army or Vietnam.

It was a shocker to those of us who had thought we'd been spared. I had my orders to Japan, while others had orders for medical facilities and hospitals in Germany, England, Korea, Okinawa, the Middle East, and the Philippines. For all of us, it meant another year wherever we were going, but a year that would keep us safely out of the war zone.

A bit elitist and definitely pampered throughout college as pre-med students, and admired throughout medical school as future physicians, we all pretty much expected to do what we wanted, or at least be listened to when it came to things we thought were important. None of us expected to be told what to do by someone who wasn't a physician, much less someone who probably had never finished college.

Not to be asked what we wanted and without so much as a minimal negotiation, simply because someone else wanted it done their way, left all of us stunned. Again, we'd missed that one, too. Clearly, an organization dedicated to killing people and breaking things was not fundamentally subtle or willing to give any view other than their own much consideration.

The twenty-four hours following that ultimatum remain confusing and mysterious to this day, both to me and to everyone else having been given that Hobson's choice. Surprisingly though, there was no glee or sense of smugness on the part of those in the class who had come to basic training already going to 'Nam. Almost the whole class was now in the same boat. Apparently, at least in some cases, envy is not mean-spirited. That, too, was a surprise.

The truth was that the new orders made those who were already headed to 'Nam even grimmer. The real message to them was that this shifting about of personnel meant that, with more doctors needed in 'Nam, things were clearly going even worse than the Army was willing to admit.

It definitely was not a good sign for anyone already going to 'Nam, whether soldier, special forces, marine, or physician. That, coupled to the military's strange view of modern medicine, made the ultimatum seem even more bizarre and more dangerous. It didn't really matter to the Army what kind of doctor you were or how well-trained you'd been in your specialty. In the end, to the Army, a doctor was a doctor and all of us should be able, regardless of training or sub-specialty, to keep a wounded soldier alive.

It was at best an old-fashioned view of medicine and one that seemed to all of us not only archaic, but suicidal. But forget about democracy or reason and maybe even the truth in the military. This was the Army's game, and they were in charge. They could do what they wanted. That, too, was a surprise for the naïve among us.

By that evening, the shock at the ultimatum had turned to a kind of silent outrage. Everyone who had a family member who knew anyone in government, from congressmen and senators to state representatives, made calls. If it wasn't panic, it was close.

"Unfair" … "Stupid" … "Astonishingly short-sighted" … "What good am I going to be in a Battalion Aid Station when I have my boards in Gastroenterology?"

But in private, thoughts were, "What about my family? Who is going to take care of them if I get killed?" "They're treating me like I'm some eighteen-year-old school kid." "I'm not going to be much good to anyone not practicing what I've been trained to do."

And then came the real anger and sense of abuse. "This wasn't the deal we were given." "Hell, if I knew this would happen I'd have gone into the Army right after medical school and gotten the two years of military service over with once and for all."

No one said what was really on his mind, the "What about me?" And that was pretty much what I thought too: "What about me?" But I already knew how this would all turn out from that Pentagon letter to the chief of my hospital. There was a war going on.

The Army was in charge. In the end, everyone who went in to see the major extended, but me. I was one of the few single physicians in our class. No family, no kids, no responsibilities. Before I left for the Army, I had sold my Volvo and put what little I owned into a few boxes and left them in the basement of the home of one of the staff physicians at the county hospital to be stored until I came back to the States.

I had left for Fort Sam without owning anything and without having a single key in my pocket. There were no excuses I could use, except the excuse of being afraid. Caving into that seemed a bad precedent for the future. Besides, giving the Army three years of my life seemed a very long time, as well as a very bad deal. I did want to get on with things. Extending would clearly have been worth it if I were to be killed or wounded. But in the end, time won out. I guess I still didn't know enough, back then, to do the right and prudent thing.

The next afternoon, I walked into the major's office and told him that I would not extend. Instead, I'd go to Vietnam. As soon as I said it, I knew it had all been a scam. It actually took the major a few seconds to look up from my personnel file. There was more of a look of confusion on his face than surprise.

The major and the Army had been bluffing. And why wouldn't they try to get the best deal they could? When you thought about it, the military had bases all over the world and needed doctors where they had always needed them—everywhere. Getting another twelve months of active duty out of two or three hundred physicians a year was a real bonus. The Army had nothing to lose, so why not try?

The major though, clearly unprepared for my answer, quickly began to backtrack as he started to look through my papers. "Well," he said, trying to get back in control, "You are single." Not looking up, he continued to look through the file, "and that extra year in Japan would allow you to have an accompanied tour … but in your case," he added as if talking to himself, "that really wouldn't make much sense."

I didn't know if that was a question or an answer. The major did take one last shot at it. "Are you sure?" he asked, finally looking up. "I mean, Japan can be a pretty nice tour of duty for a single guy." He left out the part about not getting killed or wounded.

I learned the next day that everyone else in our Basic Training Class, as in most of the other classes, had extended for that extra year. The Army was true to its word. Everyone who extended did keep his original permanent duty station and did get an accompanied tour.

To this day, I still don't know how many physicians were killed or wounded in 'Nam. What I do know is that none of the physicians who extended was among the casualties. From what I was to learn over the next two years, staying that extra year in Germany or Korea or the Philippines didn't seem to have been such a bad idea.

I went to the Army Hospital at Camp Zama, Japan for the usual two years of military duty, where, quite surprisingly, the war found me. It was four weeks after I arrived at Zama that the military command in Vietnam sent the 101st Airborne back again into the Ashow Valley. They were mauled, killed, and wounded in that tall elephant grass, with the survivors quickly med-evaced to the nearest surgical hospitals and from the surgical hospitals to us at Zama.

3.

ZAMA / THE WOUNDED

If basic training for physicians at Fort Sam had been the Cliff's Notes for taking care of the casualties of Vietnam, Zama was the real thing. Before the Vietnam War, Zama had been no more than a 90-bed Army dispensary, a hold-over from the Korean War. In fact, there was little else in military medical facilities in all the rest of Southeast Asia. When President Johnson listened to his military advisers and sent in ground troops to replace the advisers that Kennedy had approved a few years earlier, the military had the choice of expanding the existing medical facilities in Japan, building up those in the Philippines, or starting from scratch in Okinawa. Okinawa was too expensive. The Philippines looked a bit too unstable. So, the Army chose Japan.

The dispensary at Zama was quickly upgraded to a large general hospital. The Vietnam evacs came in through the large U.S. Air Force base at Yokota, a few minute's helicopter flight time from Zama. Over the years, smaller specialty hospitals with additional capabilities—neurosurgical, burns, and orthopedic—were built in an arc around Zama throughout the Kanto Plains surrounding Tokyo.

I had no idea how the Kanto plains looked before the war. At one time, it must have been a pretty place. There were woodblock prints from the Mejia on the walls of the Officer's

Club at Zama that showed the plains tranquil and lovely, nestled comfortably at the foot of the mountains.

But there was little beauty there when I arrived. Like the wounds, the rivers ran, polluted and ugly, from a dirty green to a metallic gray; the rice and barley fields that used to be there had been replaced by square, filthy factories. Even the air smelled; every day was like living behind a Mexican bus. Still, no one was shooting at you here. There were no ambushes or hunter-killer teams. No one was sending out the LRRPs (Long Range Reconnaissance Patrols) and at night you couldn't hear them pounding in mortar tubes across the rivers. That was something. You could see it on the faces of the troopers they carried in off the choppers. It didn't matter to them that the place smelled or that the smoke from Yokahama and Yokuska blotted out the stars. All that counted was that their war was over for awhile and they had gotten out alive.

It didn't take any of us any time to figure out how it really worked. The casualties stayed overnight at the 20th casualty staging area at Yokota, where they were stabilized. They were checked by the docs and nurses, re-hydrated if necessary, had their wounds looked at, bandages changed, and their pain medications adjusted.

'Nam is always hot, sometimes 110 in the shade, and most of the casualties had been humping it for days. There might have been half a million men in Vietnam by 1968, but only about 100,000 did the fighting. You didn't see much combat as a clerk typist sitting in Saigon or a supply sergeant in Cam Ran Bay. Those who did the fighting were fighting all the time.

The fluids these kids would get at the 20th did give them the edge. If they were critical or just seriously ill and the decision was made that they couldn't wait, they'd be med-evaced by chopper as soon as they got off the C-141s to Zama or one of the other three hospitals.

There was once a tennis court at Zama, out near the administration building. During the Tet Offensive, the fence had been torn down and the asphalt used for another helipad. Apparently, no one had thought or even considered putting back the fence.

30

It was simply understood that the tennis court stayed a landing pad. Maybe those in charge were not expecting another Tet, but neither where they expecting the war to end any time soon. At least that much was clear from the very moment I arrived from the States.

And this is how it worked for the 58,264 who would be killed and the 350,000 who would be wounded. This was Vietnam and this was military medicine that was, in fact, 1968 civilian trauma medicine brought to the battlefield. The difference of course was the medics. Not many city ambulance drivers or EMTs would have to run through machine gun fire to get to the wounded. But that happened all the time in 'Nam. It happened so often that the VC and NVA would hit the point on a patrol and try not to kill him but to get him screaming for help and then they would get the medic too. He'd come, they knew he would.

And it is the same in Iraq and Afghanistan. The Iraqi insurgents and the Afghan Taliban will set their explosives to kill or wound as many soldiers and marines as they can, but they will also put out secondary charges to get the medics who, they too are sure, will come. The two enemies—even decades apart—would rather wound our troops than kill them. If you are dead, you are dead. But to be wounded means that others in your squad or platoon have to give up the fight to take care of you and if possible carry you to safety or at least out of the fight. It is always better to wound the enemy in a firefight than to kill them.

Back then, the Army prided itself that anyone hit was no more than ten minutes away from the nearest surgical or evac hospital. Technically, they were right. But like so much in the military, then as now, they weren't quite accurate. Once a dust-off did pick you up, it was usually a ten-minute flight to the nearest surgical or evac hospital, maybe a little longer if you were really lit up and the chopper had to overfly the nearest surgical facility and go on to the closest evac hospital. But the choppers still had to get in and get the wounded troopers out. By the time I got to Zama, over 3,000 choppers had been shot down and more than one medic had to watch the wounded die because they'd run out of plasma and couldn't be resupplied, or the med-evac couldn't get in to pick up the casualty. Basically, the wounded bled to death. And that happened a lot. If there was anything positive that came out of the "shock and awe" of Vietnam, it was the advances in vascular surgery that were pushed forward by the large number of high velocity wounds, with their vascular and organ damage, that happened on the battlefields of Southeast Asia.

But if you were alive by the time the medic got to you and certainly if you were still alive by the time they managed to stop the bleeding, start an IV for some blood or plasma, and managed to put you on the chopper, you'd most likely live. And that is what happened a lot of the time and that is what the medics were trained to do. In a very real way what the medics did was little more than Boy Scout stuff, but at the time so was a great deal of medicine itself, especially surgery. In the late 1960s, surgeons were still doing radical mastectomies for breast cancer while hip replacements were just being developed in England.

Vascular surgery in the form of coronary by-pass was beginning to come into its own, while the first dialysis machines—the size of grand pianos—were being fitted with wheels to be used in intensive care units. There were no CT scans or MRIs available in any X-ray departments anywhere, and no antibiotics to treat resistant staph infections, and nobody had any idea what was causing Toxic Shock Syndrome, Lupus, Scleroderma, or Multiple Sclerosis.

But there were concentrated blood volume expanders, and with the advances in vascular surgery, the ability to suture up torn blood vessels and put in blood vessel grafts, along with a growing understanding of the physiology of shock and blood loss. All that was to come together in the jungles and rice paddies of Vietnam, Laos, and Cambodia, as it did in the trauma centers in our largest cities.

In all major traumatic injuries, whether during an ambush along a trail in the Mekong Delta, a firefight in the Central Highlands, a motorcycle or a car accident on a major U.S. freeway, what kills you is blood loss. Bleeding from a penetrating chest wound or an abdominal injury, unless the bleeding can be stopped, is universally fatal. It has always been that way. Indeed, when Alexander Hamilton was shot in the abdomen by Aaron Burr, he told the physician in attendance at the duel that "this is a mortal wound." And it was. Hamilton had bled to death by the next afternoon.

But if the bleeding can be stopped with compression, a surgical pack, or the use of a tourniquet or a clamp, and if you could get some blood or plasma and pain medications to deal with the developing shock in a timely fashion—and then get to a hospital for a more definitive and if necessary reconstructive surgery where damaged organs can be removed or sutured, and blood vessels either grafted or tied off—usually within an hour of being wounded on a battlefield or injured in an accident on a freeway—you'll most likely survive.

In modern trauma medicine, it's called the "golden hour." And that's what the medics did in 'Nam. They tried, and many times succeeded, in keeping the wounded alive through that golden hour. They packed wounds, gave injections of morphine, put on tourniquets, carried needles to start IVs in order to hang bottles of plasma and when they had to—and only if they had to—cut open the neck to do an in-the-field tracheotomy in order to clear the airway of blood and keep the injured soldier or marine breathing, or at least give them the chance to keep breathing until they could make it to a chopper.

There would be a difference in our next two big wars, Iraq and Afghanistan. There would be fewer deaths and more brain and extremity injuries. Our wars of bleeding to death would be over and in their place were amputations and traumatic brain injuries. The difference would not only be the result of different weapons and a better understanding of the biochemical and physiologic effects of severe trauma to the human body, but more effective body armor.

A large part of what would become a rather astonishing 16 casualties to every death in Iraq and Afghanistan against the 2.4 casualties to deaths in Vietnam would have to do with the development of effective body armor. There was a kind of body armor in Vietnam. They were flack vests that protected the chest, along with the heart and major blood vessels going to the lungs, brain, and abdomen. But the vests were heavy and the armor plates within the vest did not cover all the areas of the upper torso, leaving spaces between the vests and the body as well as between the plates. And 'Nam is hot and wearing a twenty-pound vest while carrying a full pack and having to hump it for miles through dense humid jungle was simply not considered to be worth the effort or the discomfort, especially since those vests didn't always work.

The gaps in the vests left areas of the chest unprotected and the soldiers and marines could clearly see the immediate and overall results, especially when the vests were hit by a 30-caliber round fired from a few yards away or a 50-caliber round fired from anywhere. The steel plates themselves could be pierced. In short, the vests did not cover enough of the body and they did not stop the fully jacketed AK-47 rounds, and for the most part didn't protect soldiers from mortars, anti-personnel mines, or shrapnel wounds.

But looking back at it now, maybe it was because these kids were all draftees and so didn't view themselves as professionals, or maybe it was because the vests didn't work all the time, or maybe it was just the heat, or maybe it was simply easier to forget about any kind of protection and hope for the best. It was probably all four. Vietnam was that kind of place.

But all that changed by October 7, 2001, when U.S. forces entered Afghanistan to destroy Al Qaeda and defeat the Taliban. A significant part of Iraq's and Afghanistan's astonishing survival rates began there in the mountains of Tora Bora.

Today's armor is made of a combination of ceramic plates and Kevlar. The new vests are lighter and more flexible than the 1960s Vietnam-era vests, and they cover more of the trunk and torso. During the search for Osama Bin Laden, a Special Forces trooper in the mountain ranges of the tribal areas of West Afghanistan was shot at close range. Rounds from an AK-47 hit him in the chest. The trooper dropped to the ground, but a few moments later rose up to shoot and kill his attacker.

According to those who were there, it was like seeing Lazarus rise from the dead. Only this Lazarus rose up with an M-4 still in his hand. It was something that simply had never happened in any other war. Today's more effective body armor, which better protects the chest, heart, lungs, back, and upper abdomen, is a major part of the new survivability. But both our country and our casualties have paid an unexpected and unanticipated price for enduring as well as surviving.

In a way, we have been lulled by our own successes in simply keeping our troops alive—as if death is the only measure of risks on the battlefield—into a strange kind of reverie. Despite the growing sophistication of our battlefield medicine and the new body armor, the orthopedic wards at Walter Reed are becoming filled with numbers of multiple amputees not seen since the Civil War. The wounded are being admitted to the surgical hospitals with a new diagnosis of "polytrauma" for those with brain, muscle, skin, and extremity injuries. More and more beds are being added as well to the neurosurgery units, and the ortho-pedics wards, with longer waits in the rehabilitation and PTSD clinics of the VA hospitals. What has changed in these new wars is that our troops are now being blown up rather than just shot.

But back in Vietnam, the medics did manage to keep those they could alive, in order to get them to the surgical hospitals, and the surgical hospitals fixed what they could, in order to pass them on to the evac hospitals, who sent them on to us in Japan, where our job was to finally fix what could be fixed, in order to finally get them home.

But getting them home could take quite some time, and even with that, we might not be sending them back exactly the same as when they'd been sent to 'Nam. Still, we tried, and did the best we could, but it wasn't like today and medicine wasn't all that sophisticated.

There wasn't a great deal that we could do to make things right in the late 1960s. Lower extremity prosthetic devices, unlike the devices of today, gave only support, while the upper extremity prosthetic devices were little more than hooks. There were no intra-cranial monitors and the numbers of available antibiotics were limited, in the face of more complicated and difficult to treat infections.

'Nam, besides being hot, was a very dirty place where most of the wounds were contaminated, if not when the troopers were hit, then as they were carried through the clouds of dust and dirt raised by the rotor blades of the med-evac choppers as the engines were feathered to be ready for a rapid take off.

Eventually, but usually within days, the majority of surgeries at Zama became no more than cutting out what had finally become clear was dead, needed to be removed, or involved taking off what was no longer, or would never be, functional, and then kind of sitting back and hoping for the best. Compared to today, it was a patchwork kind of medicine, but if we could beat the infections and handle the major organ system damage, we would be able to get them home.

The survival rate for those who were carried off the choppers at Zama was over 98 percent. Even those who should have died would surprise us by somehow managing to survive. We took pride and comfort in that much. But it wasn't easy. I remember one of the soldiers the plastic surgeons had kept for the whole time I was at Zama. He was there the day I arrived and was still there the day I left. They couldn't do what the plastic surgeons can do now, so they kept him as they tried multiple and painful reconstructions to rebuild his face, which had literally been blown away by an exploding RPG. All of today's minimally invasive techniques and laser surgeries, along with the use of synthetic polymers for structural reconstructions, were decades off. So with the initial results not going that well, the surgeons simply kept him at Zama.

Over the years that I was there, the face did get better, or at least more recognizable as a face, or we simply got used to seeing what was there and thought that, all things considered, it was going pretty well. With more surgeries and additional skin flaps followed by even more reconstructions of his mouth and nose, and then his lips and eye lids, with the passage of time, we thought that he did look better, though we feared that when he would finally be sent home someone would either look away, or be foolish enough to ask what had happened to him.

And then there was Max Cleland, a young lieutenant in the First Air Cav who was later—much later—to become the junior Senator from Georgia. He was not only one of those survivors who made it to the med-evac chopper, but in many ways the poster boy for Vietnam, for the evac chain, for Zama, for both the stupidity and confusion of the war as well as all the courage, suffering, and bravery.

I remember seeing Max in the intensive care unit, his still-oozing stumps up on blocks, his left arm completely gone at the shoulder, tubes running into his chest and what remained of his abdomen. His story, like so many stories in 'Nam, was simple enough.

The First Air Cavalry had begun to chopper in troops to replace the Marines who had put up a three-month-long resistance against North Vietnamese regulars during the battle for Khe Sanh in the northern Central Highlands of Vietnam.

The Marines had survived dozens of assaults, constant mortar and artillery fire, and a whole host of frontal attacks. Finally, after enduring enough casualties from B-52 raids and hundreds of fighter-bomber sorties along with their tons of high explosives, white phosphorous, and napalm, the North Vietnamese simply gave up and disappeared back into the jungle. In reality, the Marines had survived on our immense firepower and the fact that our military would not let the base be overrun. But it had been a very close call.

Two companies of the First Air Cavalry were to be the Marines' replacement. Max, a Southerner with political ambitions, had volunteered for the military first as an American, second as a Southerner, and third as a potential politician who had been told by his mentors in Georgia that a military background could not hurt an aspiring politician. You do make your choices and you do take your consequences.

The story of the loss of both his legs and his left arm and parts of his lower abdomen has become a bit confused over the years. What we heard when he first arrived at Zama was that when he was jumping out of the chopper at Khe Sanh, a grenade clipped to his web gear got caught on one of the door jambs and the pin was pulled as he left the open doorway.

Either he'd forgotten or hadn't been in 'Nam long enough to learn that you have to tape down the lever arm on your grenades, or you run the risk of the pin inadvertently being pulled out as you moved through the jungle or, in Max's case, as you exited a chopper.

Apparently Max was able to get his web gear down around his knees before the grenade exploded.

There were discussions among the surgeons and the nurses as to whether or not it might be better to just let him die. But he survived and eventually was sent on to Walter Reed, and after a few years at Reed he went back home to Georgia.

Three decades later, the story changed when a trooper, on the same chopper as Max, came forward. He said that he was behind Max in the chopper when they both jumped out of the doorway and that he had dropped a grenade that he was holding in his hand when he'd hit the ground. It was his grenade that had rolled forward and blew up under Max. So it wasn't really Max's fault. It was the stupidity or carelessness of war itself. I am sure that the new explanation for the loss of his three limbs was of some comfort to Max. Heaven knows there was little enough comfort for anyone in that war. But that was what Vietnam was like—filled with confusing stories, outright lies, terrible decisions, bizarre unexplainable and unexpected results, distortions of the truth, foolishness, stupidity, courage, bravery, and in more cases than anyone would be willing to admit, a kind of dazzling grace. And nowhere was that grace more clearly seen than in the medics.

4.

THE MEDICS / THEN AND NOW

Who do you ask if there is a disaster? If there is a tornado in Alabama you don't ask the people in Florida what happened ...

—Conversation: Wounded Medic, Surgical Ward,
Camp Zama, Japan

Back in late 1969, *Life Magazine* had a pictorial covering the medical evacuation chain, from the battlefields of Vietnam through the battalion aid stations, all the way to Japan, and from Japan on to the States. For some reason that still baffles me, and it certainly surprised every physician in the military who saw the magazine, the editors and photographers of *Life* had picked a young white officer, as I remember a college graduate from some eastern university, with a minor hand wound. It might have hurt. You could see that much on the face of the young lieutenant in the photograph as they carried him off the chopper. But it definitely wasn't reality.

The country clearly had no idea what was really going on then, anymore than it knows what is going on now. If *Life Magazine* was willing to present fiction as fact, then there was truly no way out of the mess. It would just go on forever. I remembered thinking about why the editors hadn't picked someone with a penetrating head wound, a transected spinal cord, or no face? I understood, as did everyone else at Zama, or at the Burn Ward at

Kishine, or the Neurosurgery Unit at Drake, that this war was a lot more ferocious than anyone was willing to admit, much less acknowledge, and a lot more devastating than a hand wound.

What happened in Vietnam and what was presented in *Life Magazine* as the truth has been trumped by an even more insidious silence, or rather disinterest, for both Iraq and Afghanistan. We don't have pictures of any kind of injury. For our latest wars there are not even pictures allowed of caskets coming home, the C-5As that bring the wounded in from Iraq and Afghanistan have been ordered to land at Dover Air Force Base in Delaware only at night. Our past President did not attend military funerals, and there was a moratorium on medals given out for courage and bravery, as if to downplay the dangers as well as the desperateness of the fighting. What is hoped for is that out of sight will be out of mind. And for the most part the silences have worked. We were told to just go shopping and basically to leave the fighting and the wars to someone else.

The truth was that back in Vietnam, no one, including the editors of *Life Magazine,* was seeing the whole thing. Vietnam, like all wars, came in pieces. In a very real way, everyone saw only their part of it, and that alone made it easy to dismiss what was really important. You could see what you wanted and parse whatever you saw any number of ways and no one could really say you were wrong. It was the old "You were given the wrong information"... "You didn't get the full picture"... "You talked to the wrong people"... "You don't understand the long-term goals" ... "You're not a team player"... "Give it a chance, it will work."

But it did seem to me at the time that if you really wanted to know the true costs of a disaster, you had better ask those really involved, and better still, those actually paying the price. And those were clearly the ones I saw at Zama, and today those landing at Dover, and the ones being carried off the med-evac C-5 at Andrews yesterday, today, and tomorrow.

So, *Life Magazine* aside, I realized after a month or two at Zama that the whole war was coming to me and not just the war, but the price we were paying for that war. Out of those two years came the book *365 Days,* which was nominated for The National Book Award. But back then, what I found baffling, and still today find so amazing, is that what I discovered and wrote down that was actually taking place, was during the time when we were all reading in the stateside newspapers that America was going to hell and that it was impossible to get an American teenager to act responsibly, listen to authority, to do what was asked, or for that matter to care about anyone but themselves.

You would have thought then that it would be a hopeless task to get them to kill themselves for something as vague as duty, or to run through mortars and machine gun fire for anything as subtle as concern. But during the first five hours of what was to be called "Hamburger Hill," fifteen medics were hit and ten were killed. There was not one medic left standing. The 101st had to bring in combat assault medics from two other companies during the firefight and by nine that night, every one of those medics too, had been killed or wounded.

At the time, the Army psychiatrists at Zama called it a simple matter of roles. Soldiers and marines fight and die for each other, while medics growing up in the hypocritical adult world of Salinger's Holden Caulfield, and placed at the heart of a war that even the dullest of them eventually found difficult to believe in, much less die for, were suddenly tapped, not for their selfishness or greed, but for their grace and wisdom, not for their brutality, but for their love and concern. The medic begins after a very short time to think of himself as a doctor as well as a savior. The fact that the units returned the medic's concern with their own wholehearted respect and affection made the whole thing work. In a world of suffering and death, Vietnam became a Walt Disney true-life adventure, where the young were suddenly left alone to care for the young.

That was then...

Graham was eighteen years old when a tracer round skidded off his flack vest and triggered a grenade in his webbing. He struggled for a moment to pull it off and then, according to the other medic working with him, he jumped out of the aid station, and kept running, with the grenade bouncing against his chest until it went off.

Webb had been in 'Nam only three days when he got into his first firefight. The 3rd Platoon working out ahead had killed three dinks near a bridge. A few hundred meters farther they found a small arms cache with four AK-50s, a couple of RPDs, and a Smirnov attack rifle. They waited for the rest of the company and then they all moved out through the waist-high grass. You could feel trouble coming; up and down the line, the troopers switched their weapons to automatic and shifted their rucksacks so they could drop them more easily. The machine gunners began carrying their weapons at port arms instead of across their shoulders. The grenadiers loaded their M-79s with canister rounds. Up ahead, fifty meters away, was a thick tree line. The only sound was the company moving through the grass and an occasional tinkle of loose gear. Webb was walking with the Sergeant.

"Thirty meters," the Sergeant said softly, "we'll get hit inside of thirty meters."

"Sooner," a trooper offered drily. Twenty meters farther, the firing began. Even as he hit the ground, Webb saw three figures tumble over in front of him. Within seconds, the whole field was exploding. Automatic fire cracked and snapped through the dry grass. An RPD hidden off to the right began firing and caught a squad trying to move off that way. Two other machine guns opened up on the left. Seeing where they were falling, the VC began skipping rounds into them.

Behind and overhead, Webb could hear the gunships thumping their way toward them. The Vietnamese stopped firing as the first loach, small and agile, swept in over their heads. A moment later, a Cobra swung in. Everybody was popping smoke grenades. Webb got to his knees and, seeing a trooper dragging a body toward a nearby rise, shook off his rucksack. Taking his helmet off and leaving it on the ground with his M-16, he got to his feet and began running toward them with his aid kit. He made ten meters before they got him: a clean straight round that caught him under his swinging left arm and came out the other side of his chest.

This is now...

Johnson was twenty-two years old when the firefight broke out. It started with an IED that disabled one of the Humvees, killing the driver and severely wounding the machine gunner. The IED blast was followed by an attack where a dozen Taliban began to fire at the platoon from across an orchard. Two more marines were hit and dragged behind one of the stone walls near the road. Johnson picked up the medical kit and started to sprint towards the wall when a round hit him in the neck. Unable to stop the bleeding, he was dead a few minutes later—

5.

AMERICA'S WARS / AN AUTOPSY REPORT

We rely on things, an enormous number of things. In the Second World War there were B-17s and B-24s, B-26s and B-29s, along with P-38 Lightings and P-51 Mustangs. The Navy had over thirty-six different kinds of ships in its fleet firing over two dozen different guns of some twenty different calibers. Our army went ashore at Normandy with dozens of types of trucks and tanks. Over 1,667 tons of bombs were dropped by 279 B-29s in one night, causing the firestorm of Tokyo that led to the destruction of over 300,000 buildings and approximately 125,000 deaths. And of course there were our atomic bombs.

There are military historians who have commented that our ultimate victory in World War II was not so much a victory based on tactics and strategy as it was on the unfolding industrial might of the United States. General Fred C. Weyand, Chief of Staff of the Army, in his 1976 analysis of the Vietnam War said much the same thing, though in decidedly starker terms:

War is Death and Destruction. The American way of war is particularly violent, deadly and dreadful. We believe in using "things"—artillery, bombs, massive firepower—-in order to conserve our soldiers' lives. The enemy, on the other hand, makes up for his lack of "things" by expending men instead of machines, and for that suffers enormous casualties. The Army saw this happening in

Korea, and we should have made the realities of [the Vietnam War] obvious to the American people before they witnessed it on their television screens. The Army must make the price of involvement clear before we get involved ...

Nowhere is this understanding of technical and industrial power as an element of winning our wars more dramatically and clearly explained than during the questioning of an unrepentant captured German officer by an American captain following the breakthrough of the German lines surrounding the 101st Airborne at Bastogne during the Battle of The Bulge in late 1945. Clearly irritated by what he considered the arrogance of the German officer, the captain challenged the German that if the Wehrmacht was such a superior fighting force, what were he and his men doing in an American prisoner-of-war camp? The Germans earlier in the war had used their own technology, advanced equipment, and industrial might in the form of Ju-87 Stuka dive bombers and Tiger Tanks to win their own victories. They understood the advantages of "things".

"Well," the officer answered in perfect English, "We set up our guns. And you Americans sent a tank down the road and we destroyed it. Then you sent another tank down the same road and we destroyed that tank. Then you sent a third and fourth tank that we destroyed. Unfortunately, we ran out of ammunition before you Americans ran out of tanks."

The German officer's professional arrogance was appropriate and in a way accurate, but his unit had been defeated and he was taken prisoner, whatever the reasons. Still, a post-World War II study documented that when Americans fought the German Army, if troop numbers were equivalent on each side, the Germans, despite having less and inferior equipment, often won or inflicted a disproportionate number of Allied casualties.

But our reliance on things didn't work all that well in Korea. Despite round-the-clock artillery barrages, the Chinese were willing to take enormous casualties as they drove the Eighth Army and the First Marine Division back from the Chosin Reservoir all the way down the North Korean Peninsula into South Korea. There were reports that some units of the Chinese Army attacked with only pitchforks and axes. It was only the daily strafing runs by U.S. fighter planes that kept enough soldiers and marines alive to allow what were left of the First Marine Division and the Eighth Army back to the safety of South Korea.

Still that reliance on things continued on into Vietnam. Only then it was B-52s, C-130s, F-105s, and F-86 sabers, and helicopters, lots and lots of helicopters. There were gunships and slicks, med-evacs and Cobras, loaches and the twin engine Chinooks. And yet, after ten years of fighting with 58,000 of our own troops killed and another 400,000 wounded, we had to pack up and go home.

There is a recorded conversation held in Hanoi during the peace negotiations preceding our withdrawal from Southeast Asia: "You do know," explained an American officer to the Vietnamese negotiator, "that you never defeated us on the battlefield."

The North Vietnamese colonel pondered the remark for a moment. "That may be so," he answered carefully, "but it is also irrelevant."

If Korea was the template of what can truly happen in a poorly thought-out war, where wishful thinking and industrial might replaces reality, Vietnam became the poster-child for the rest of the Twentieth Century and the beginnings of the Twenty-first.

Senior Lieutenant Colonel Nguyen Hu An, Deputy Commander of the B-3 Front and Commanding Officer of the 66th North Vietnam Regiment explained his professional assessment of our war in an interview thirty years after the first major battle between regular forces of the North Vietnamese Army and the technologically-advanced United States Air Mobile First Air Cavalry using the new tactics of vertical envelopment.

The battle occurred deep in the Ia Drang Valley in the forested jungles of the Central Highlands near the Cambodian border during the second week in November of 1965. More than 234 troopers of the First Air Cav were killed and more than 250 wounded during the four days of the battle. The North Vietnamese paid a much higher price of over 3,500 killed and an unknown number wounded.

We had never fought the Americans and were curious about this use of helicopters, which our troops, because of the thumping noise, called tractors with propellers. During the battle, I sat out on the mountain and watched how the helicopters and aircraft were used in this new kind of war. It was very interesting.

What Colonel Hu An quickly grasped was that the North Vietnamese forces could not match the massive firepower of the Americans. He understood that any prolonged battle with the Americans, who could bring in ever-increasing fire power in the form of long-range artillery, helicopter gunships, napalm, fighter-bombers, and saturation B-52 raids, would always tip the scale of victory in their direction, no matter how hard or how bravely the North Vietnamese fought.

Colonel Hu An and other Vietnamese officers realized that the only way their units could survive a firefight, much less a battle, with the Americans was to get in close and "grab the Americans by the belt buckle," and not let go. It was clear that to give up distance during an attack or firefight was in essence to lose the battle. The strategy and the tactics would have to be to get in close and stay close, whatever the initial costs.

What the Vietnamese had learned would become painfully clear over the remaining years of the Vietnam War. The American units might pound them, but the Vietnamese could—by picking the time and place of their battles—get in close to offset the offensive firepower and then withdraw as quickly as possible after initial contacts. This made up for being outgunned, while bleeding the Americans at their own game.

All of this was, of course, not so much a way to win as it was a way not to lose. That was no small thing when the only other alternative was simply to take the pounding and die in place. But for the Vietnamese, the war was not to be a sprint, but a marathon.

It was a desperate policy, but in the give-and-take of war, it worked. Quick attacks, close-in ambushes, the breaking off of contact before the gunships and fighter bombers arrived, became the North Vietnamese way of neutralizing both American technology and American firepower. And of course, the other part of the strategy was the willingness to accept both civilian and military casualties. We would lose some 58,000 soldiers and marines over the next ten years while the North Vietnamese would lose close to 2 million.

But what was of real interest to military historians were the different conclusions drawn by the North Vietnamese Government and military compared to our own Government and Pentagon about that first battle in the Ia Drang Valley. The Johnson Administration, backed by the hawks in Congress as well as the Pentagon itself, viewed what had happened on the ground as a positive; that a death rate of ten to one meant that a war of attrition would surely prove successful. The Vietnamese took a totally different view.

In Hanoi, President Ho Chi Minh and his military commanders came to the conclusion that they could eventually win the war. Senior General Vo Nguyen Giap—a school teacher who had turned military genius, defeating both the Japanese and then the French in the years following World War II—correctly understood that the helicopter was the newest and most important innovation in the war. But he also had grasped that for all their virtuosity, the use of the helicopter was not a strategy but merely a tactic—a powerful tactic to be sure—but still no more than a tactic. "We thought the Americans must have a strategy. We did. We had a strategy of people's war. You (the Americans) had only new tactics ... your helicopters ... you need decisive tactics to win a strategic victory ... if we could defeat your helicopters then we defeat your (lack of) strategy. Our goal was to win the war." In short, the Vietnamese saw nothing different in our strategy from the French. Basically, despite all our power and technological advances, we were relying only on tactics. General Giap knew that in the long term the helicopter, as well as the new technologies, would not be enough. And of course, the North Vietnamese were willing to take whatever casualties it took in order to win. Despite what the experts and even the pundits might offer, in any war the enemy does have a say in how things turn out.

General Giap wrote with uncanny insight about what would be the future course of the war:

> *The enemy will pass slowly from the offensive to the defensive. The blitzkrieg will transform itself into a war of long duration. Thus, the enemy will be caught in a dilemma: He has to drag out the war in order to win it but does not possess, on the other hand, the psychological and political means to fight a long-drawn-out war.*

At the beginning of the Iraq and Afghanistan wars, the numbers of patients suffering flashbacks who were being admitted to the PTSD clinics of the VA hospitals quadrupled. What surprised the physicians and psychologists running the clinics was that these patients were not those who had recently been deployed to Iraq and Afghanistan; they were the Vietnam veterans whose remembrances of the war had been reactivated by the deployment of a new generation of young soldiers and marines sent into what appeared to be another hopeless war set out once again at the very borders of things. But that kind of reactivated PTSD would eventually affect the whole country, if in no other way, through the personal desire not to remember and then the collective effort to simply forget.

James Kitfield, in his 1995 book, *Prodigal Soldiers: How the Generation of Officers Born of Vietnam Revolutionized the American Style of War*, deals with the years from the end of the Vietnam war to the First Gulf War in 1991. He documents the lives, ideas, and struggles of those few officers who, at great personal sacrifice and facing enormous professional and public ridicule, stayed in the military after Vietnam to reinvent and reconstitute an army and a military culture no longer crippled by the effects of that war, nor abused by those it was pledged to protect.

Those officers focused on re-establishing morale within the military, the confidence of the country in its armed forces, and a new professionalism among the officers and enlisted ranks. The "Be All You Can Be" motto came out of that era of rebuilding, as did a more defined role for committing the U.S. Army, Air Force, and Marines.

The history of our military during the late 1970s, through the 80s and 1990s was also one of refinement of tactics and force structure as much as it was strategy. The change in strategy was simple enough. The new post-Vietnam doctrine—put into place by Secretary of Defense Casper Weinberger and Secretary of State Colin Powell—insisted on no war without first putting into place overwhelming force. No war without the commitment of the whole country. No war without well-defined goals and no war without an appropriate and attainable exit strategy.

But unfortunately the operational emphasis of this transformation was again on "things." Much of the effort and focus was on increasing the lethality of weapon systems, with the blueprint for it all being a military able to defeat any army anywhere in the world. Apparently no one asked if our new enemies would actually be armies. But whoever the enemy might be, technology became the default mode for the transformation.

The Army, Air Force, Marines, and Navy developed computerized technologies to re-task combat assets in real time, and found ways to increase their strike capabilities by bringing more modern and lethal firepower to bear at those points where their new computerized programs indicated that maximum force would not only work but was an absolute requirement for success.

Colonel Douglas A. Macgregor, in his monograph *Breaking the Phalanx*, recommended a reconfiguration of combat units to ensure more mobility and flexibility, while giving those units the ability to concentrate overwhelming force at the precise time and, at what were calculated to be, the exact and necessary points of engagement. Macgregor clearly understood that as a technologically advanced and innovative nation we should use those very talents to bear on the problem of military efficiency and effectiveness.

The adaptations to what the military theorist had begun to call the new realities of both symmetrical and asymmetrical warfare were greeted with enthusiasm by the military-industrial complex only too pleased to develop the hardware to "extend the battlefield in both time and place" while giving both "increased informational awareness as well as immediate situational dominance" in the battlefields of the future. Change the vocabulary and you change the discussion.

Those officers who stayed on to implement the new strategy with the new technical advances formed the nucleus of a military that would take on and defeat Saddam Hussein's Republican Guards in less than 100 hours during the first Persian Gulf War.

Smart bombs, in the form of satellite-guided munitions, were developed that could be sent through a second floor window in a four-story building, or take out a single truck on a bridge tracked by an unmanned predator drone flown by a technician using a real-time computer and joy stick seated in a tiny air-conditioned room at Nellis Airforce Base, Nevada—some 16,000 miles away from the bridge.

There were the advanced combat optical gunsights and night-vision goggles to be used in both fog and mist, all of which were to allow smaller and faster units carrying lighter equipment and moving quickly to overcome larger and less nimble forces. There were even new computer-generated war games that clearly showed the inevitability of these newer lighter forces to win any battle, whatever the odds, by simply adding more modern and more effective technology into the mix.

Mogadishu in early 1993, with two choppers shot down by simple rocket-propelled grenades and three more damaged by small-arms fire with eighteen American soldiers killed and over a hundred wounded, was a shock to the newly transformed military. What became clear in Mogadishu was that without old-fashioned armor, and with the vulnerability of helicopters to the close-in fighting of urban warfare, a firefight was really what it had always been. It was a group of gunmen against other gunmen, fighting not only to win, but to stay alive. And in those real life gunfights, the side with the most gunmen usually wins.

And that was what happened in the streets of Mogadishu and would eventually happen in the streets of the cities and towns of Iraq and along the roads of Afghanistan. Even with half a million troops in Vietnam, we never had enough troops on the ground. The narrow streets, along with militias and the gangs of Mogadishu, should have told the military and our policy makers something new, but it didn't, since all the Pentagon did was double-down on technology.

Flushed with the increasing sophistication and lethality of our things, the concentration of enemy formations—whatever their size, configuration, or force structure—was no longer viewed as an issue. And in a way it worked, at least in 2001 and at least for a short time.

There was an incident at the beginning of what can be considered The First American/Afghan War where a single Special Forces unit, using handheld GPS locators, called in air strikes on the hundreds of Taliban fighters blocking the passes out of the northern mountains leading to the wide southern planes of Afghanistan. The tribes of the Northern Alliance that had been fighting the Taliban for almost a decade and were all too familiar with the decade-long ineffectual Russian carpet-bombing, watched as U.S. F-16s dropped satellite-guided, 500-pound bombs to within twenty-five meters of their own positions. More than one uncommitted Afghan tribal chief, having watched the precision bombing that allowed the breakout onto the plains of Afghanistan, decided on the spot that they wanted to be on the side of these new guys. It was indeed a true example of real "shock and awe."

In a way, all this has made us look too good—if not to others then certainly to ourselves—at fighting the kinds of wars we want to fight, even if they are not the wars we are given. Our weapons have become too deadly, our tanks too powerful, our bombs much more precise, and our modern personal body armor too protective. But what technology gives, technology can also hide or eventually even give away.

The last Administration did indeed take the country into Iraq in April 2003 with the world's most powerful military. It had pushed for "faster, quicker, lighter" and by extension, a cheaper force structure supported by ever more lethal "on demand" fire power. And that is precisely what it had built. The past experiences of Korea, Vietnam, and Mogadishu were clearly ignored. It was not what usually happens when governments and their military go to war—starting out by fighting the last war rather than the current one—so much as simply fighting the wars we wished to fight and were convinced we would be allowed to fight.

There were those in charge who cavalierly or foolishly felt that the most powerful nation on earth should be able to do as it chose. It has been reported that in a private conversation a Bush policymaker was heard to say that "it never hurts a great nation to throw a small nation up against the wall to let everyone else know that the great nation means business." Who said that had ignored or simply forgotten the past. The American historian Arthur Schlesinger stated as the Vietnam War began to spiral out of control that the four most dangerous words in the English language are, "This time it's different."

Colonel Macgregor acknowledged, in his latest book, *Transformation Under Fire: Revolutionizing How America Fights*, that whatever the new technical advances, there is always the need for survivability once an army is set loose on an enemy force. You cannot ever discount the unexpected and fight a war on the cheap or at a distance.

When American light infantry is armed with automatic weapons and the enemy has automatic weapons, any resistance encountered is stiff because conditions of symmetry prevail.

What Macgregor is saying is that without the availability of sufficient quantities of armored equipment to use as stable and protected weapons platforms—and even with the ability to call in air assets—lightly-armed units moving through enemy territory are always in danger.

Macgregor goes on to make the statement that whatever the situation, "When significant armor arrives on the scene, the battle ends quickly." Yet, this ability to endure as well as survive was not only ignored but dismissed as unimportant by those who took us into Iraq and have now taken us back into Afghanistan.

For well over a decade now, our light infantry has been sent out in under-armored transport vehicles to fight light infantry. And the increasing deaths and increasing casualties have documented the obvious. We now have Poly-trauma Units in our VA hospitals for a reason.

In any war, weaknesses soon become apparent and those weaknesses are exploited, whether it is in Vietnam, Mogadishu, Iraq, or Afghanistan. We have a military that could level any city in the world in a few days and cripple or destroy any division of enemy troops caught out in the open within hours. Yet, our latest two wars have taken both our soldiers and our marines to the edge of the abyss. Unfortunately, while no one was looking, these are no longer the wars we wish to fight. In villages and cities and along highways and roads where quick and painless success was assured, our troops, inadequately protected, spread too thin, only partially armored, overworked and worn down, are paying the price.

General Weyand ends his 1976 analysis on *Military Tactics and Strategies* by offering the following advice:

As military professionals, we must speak out, we must counsel our political leaders and alert the American people that there is no such thing as a "splendid little war." There is no such thing as a war fought on the cheap.

The General wasn't speaking to those who had been in Vietnam, nor was he speaking to the families of those repeatedly being deployed to the Middle East, nor to those who have already made the fight in Iraq or are currently on patrol up in the mountains or on the plains of Afghanistan. He was talking to all of us.

6.

Med-evacs and Gunships / A Short and Deadly Technical History

It was true that unlike the French, who lost a whole army in Vietnam, we might have lost a platoon and even a company in an afternoon, and maybe a battalion by nightfall, but never a regiment and definitely not a division, and certainly, we would never have lost a whole army. You cannot mass against gunships or charge through mini-guns. Our slicks and gunships, loaches and Chinooks always kept us in the war and may well have kept us in Vietnam forever. But for all their versatility—the ability to overfly areas open to ambushes, to be able to get the wounded to hospitals in a timely fashion, to level areas the size of football fields with rockets and automatic fire, to deliver more troops to the battlefield while at the same time being able to bring in supplies and ammunition to units running low on both—they were very complicated machines with all kinds of mechanical problems that made them easy to shoot down. Whatever else can be said about helicopters, they are strangely fragile affairs.

Even the tiny, glass-domed loaches that could hover motionless fifteen feet off the ground and pour machine-gun fire through the six-inch slit of a pill box, or slowly and maliciously track a man down a narrow jungle path, looked out of place in the air. Helicopters have none of the grace of an airplane and even less of the style. They seem to have to tug themselves off the ground.

And once in the air they stay there, churning on through the sheer power of their engines. If anything happens to that power, and it didn't take much in Vietnam and in Mogadishu, it doesn't take much in Iraq and even less in Afghanistan …

In a very real way, we paid a deadly price for this new technology. By late 1972, more than 4,000 helicopters had been shot down. A third of all the chopper pilots who had ever been to Vietnam would be killed, wounded, or medically boarded out of the Army. The average life span of any loach pilot, whether in 'Nam, Laos, or Cambodia, was somewhere around three months. Living any longer than that was no more than sheer luck. If you weren't killed when you were shot down, you died when you crashed. The nasty little secret about choppers is that they have to be light-weight and so they're made mostly out of aluminum and with their large gas tanks filled with jet fuel they burn when they crash. Most of the burns in Vietnam, and there were a lot of them, were the result of downed helicopters. But the warrant officers who flew those choppers continued to volunteer and they still do.

Those who chose to become warrant officers and fly choppers then, or now, are of a type—lean and tough, mechanically-oriented, obsessed with speed and daring, and incredibly brave. That too, like the medics, hasn't changed. In case we forget, this was then:

My God! One moment the chopper was there, charging in protectively across the perimeter, tail up, and the next it was gone, torn apart in a monstrous ball of flame. For a moment, the sheer unexpected violence of it all held them. Stunned, the troopers looking up from the mud, watched what was left of the chopper come hurtling headless out of the flames, a great torn piece of steel plunging blindly on across the paddy.

And it doesn't take much. A single AK round is effective up to 1,200 feet; a Russian-made 51-caliber machine gun can reach out to over 5,000. A 37-mm anti-aircraft shell is effective up to almost any height. A rocket-propelled grenade or a Stinger

Missile will most likely bring down a chopper hit at any height. In the mountains of Afghanistan, the Taliban actually shot down at the choppers.

In Vietnam though, most choppers were destroyed in the thirty feet above ground when landing or taking off. At Hunter Air Force Base and Fort Rucker, the main bases for training chopper pilots, they called it the area of translational flight, the space between hover and forward flight when the lift from the rotors is decaying and the lift from the forward flight has yet to build up. The stresses on the gear train and the rotor system are simply fantastic. If anything happens then, if a rotor went, or a round ground up the gearbox, if the hub froze, or the hydraulics fouled, there was no time to change the pitch of the blades and not enough height to allow for auto rotation. It was then and still is straight down.

"Dust Off 3, confirmed—green smoke," the Sergeant said, turning to face the choppers.

They were coming in low and quick, two of them switching from side to side to shake off the dink's aim. The first Dust Off came in right over the trees and went straight into the ground at over eighty knots. The second suddenly cut out, drifted out over the perimeter, and then, with its engines howling, quickly cut back toward the landing zone. Above the ground fighting, they could hear sledge-hammer blows as the 51's slammed through it's thin aluminum skin. The Huey sputtered a moment over them and then skidded heavily into the LZ, collapsing its landing gear. It sat tilted on its broken skid while the pilot, his adolescent face drawn tight and thin, leaned out the window and motioned for them to hurry. He kept his rotors turning while the medics, moving swiftly in the semi-darkness through the great clouds of swirling, choking dust, carried on the wounded and dying. When the Dust Off was loaded, the pilot got it light on its broken skid, lifted it a few feet off the ground, then quickly spun it around. Giving it full power, he got it moving along the ground. At about fifteen feet, it started taking fire—a dark shape moving out across an even darker sky. The troopers on the ground could see the bright greenish-blue tracers bracket it, then lose themselves as if the chopper were some kind of color damper. It kept moving along at the same height until finally out of sight, its engines sputtering, the aircraft, rising suddenly out of the jungle, drifted off to the left and was gone.

A second later, a brilliant flash of yellow-red light broke the darkness behind the NVA positions. Fifteen minutes later the gunship arrived from Qui Nhou. Over the rockets and mortars and the intermittent rattling of automatic fire, the troopers could hear the dull thudding of its turbine engine churning toward them through the ever-darkening evening sky. The NVA heard it too and stopped firing. Listening, they raised the sights on their weapons and waited.

Since Vietnam, our helicopters have been continually upgraded and improved. More powerful engines have been designed, and for greater stability in flight, stronger more flexible blades, giving the drooping effect so familiar today on all our military choppers, have replaced the older, less efficient blades. But these improvements in aerodynamics and power have come at a price, the new articulating rotor hubs are incredibly complex pieces of machinery. The intricate hinges and flaps that allow the eight-foot, 1,000 pound blades to rise and fall while they are spinning at 1,800 revolutions per minute are at best difficult to maintain, much less service. Linkages can rapidly weaken, rotors can freeze; the numerous hinges and flaps necessary to allow the blades to twist and turn continually fatigue and wear out and can be damaged by being hit by a round or a piece of shrapnel.

All the complicated physics of straight up flight are still there waiting to be unleashed by a round from an AK 47, an RPG, or the blast from a missile. At eighty knots and up at 8,000 feet that can be exactly the same as dying. Those centrifugal forces that pull at every helicopter have never disappeared and are once again becoming tragically obvious in ever-increasing numbers in the mountains of Afghanistan. That much hasn't changed.

In fact, that taking over of physics is precisely what happened in 2008 when a Chinook helicopter crashed in the mountains of Afghanistan, killing all eighteen soldiers on board. The official explanation was that the Chinook had been shot down by small arms fire. But at that height and at the distances involved as well as the obvious catastrophic failure within the helicopter, the most likely explanation was a Stinger missile.

The reason for the military stating that it was small-arms fire is obvious. The Taliban are presented as a bunch of unsophisticated tribesmen, not a sophisticated fighting force using modern weapons that put our own troops at a disadvantage. Yet, whatever the official explanation, the most likely reason for the shooting down of our helicopters in the mountains or on the plains of Afghanistan is missiles.

There was an additional startling but not unexpected fact about that Chinook. Every soldier on the chopper who died was over forty years of age. They were all National Guard troops and a number were women, some mothers and even a grandmother. We have sent our National Guard, husbands and wives, grandmothers and grandfathers, to take on the Taliban. We simply do not have, nor have we ever had, enough regular army troops to make this fight and so it is grandparents, neighbors, and friends who are getting shot down and killed.

The truth is that Afghanistan is not a very good helicopter war. Choppers do not work well at over 9,000 feet. Even with the newer more powerful engines, the air is too thin at those heights to give much lift. And in the hot summer weather the rising air is even thinner, offering less lift and less maneuverability.

And the difficult mountainous terrain with the steep canyon walls offers little opportunity for choppers to take evasive action, and so they are easily targeted and easily shot down as they enter or leave the different valleys. In some of the more remote areas, poor lift and poor maneuverability have made med-evacs difficult or simply unavailable. The choppers simply cannot get in to pick up the wounded. That so called "golden hour of survival," when bleeding can be stopped and blood and fluids given, is gone. Our marines and soldiers have to carry the wounded down off the mountaintops on stretchers. The same mountains where in the Nineteenth Century the British lost a whole army, 20,000 troops, in the Second Anglo-Afghan War. The troops were ambushed and massacred in those passes early in 1842, the wounded killed even as the few survivors tried to carried them down the mountains.

The rest of his patrol was still fighting. A Black Hawk med-evac helicopter flew above treetops towards him. Bullets cracked past. The chopper banked this way and that and hovered dangerously before landing nearby. The week before a Black Hawk on a similar med-evac mission had been shot down by a rocket-propelled grenade, and the four members of the crew had been killed. Their escort aircraft buzzed low-elevation circles around the landing area, gunners leaning out. The bullets kept coming.

If all this keeps up, we will be losing choppers in Afghanistan at rates not seen since Vietnam and, like Vietnam, the numbers of casualties will once again begin to approach the numbers of deaths. No longer will the ratio of casualties to deaths be sixteen to one but closer to two to one and three to one. That is not a virtue. A colonel in the Third Infantry Division said much the same thing early in the Iraq war when he muttered under his breath after a particularly bloody day for his troops in the Sunni Triangle, that, "Those in charge of this war have the three qualities virtually guaranteed to cause a disaster: arrogant, incompetent, and in charge."

7.

THE CHANGING FACE
OF MILITARY MEDICINE

Combat injuries have always tried the efforts of physicians and surgeons to keep a step ahead of catastrophe, not only for individuals but for armies. Swords, lances, and arrows could be lethal enough, but the use of gunpowder brought a new dimension of both death and injury to warfare. Medicine has been trying to figure it out, or at least keep ahead of this new lethality, ever since the first spears and arrows, as well as the first cannon and the first blunderbuss were fired at the beginning of the Sixteenth Century. The military barber-surgeons were startled by the extent and severity of gunshot wounds. They were most amazed at the sudden appearance of purulent drainage and the rapid spread of what was call "corruption" throughout the gun-damaged limbs and the massive abdominal and chest injuries.

The idea quickly spread that the corruption was due to the poisoning of these wounds by the gunpowder that had contaminated them and was best treated with hot oils. The treatment was to pour the hot oils into the wounds to clear out the poison. It was the practice of the day but it was very painful, adding to the misery of the patients while further damaging the surviving tissues. But even 600 years ago accepted medical practice trumped basic observation, with surgeons expected to do things, even if doing things amounted to pouring hot oil into open wounds.

It was during the 1537 campaign of Francis I in Piedmont, in the war between the French and the Holy Roman Emperor Charles over lands disputed by the King and the Emperor, that Ambroise Paré, a French surgeon, ran out of hot oil and began using only clean bandages and soaps. He quickly noticed that patients treated without the hot oils did better than the patients treated by the standard practice of the day. Paré had the temerity to trust in what he saw rather than what was taught and to advocate his new treatment against the established medical practice.

A keen observer, Paré went on to make other battlefield discoveries that led to what medical historians finally called the era of "rational surgery." Leaving aside the discovery that simply cleaning a wound was the best possible care of gunshot wounds, Paré's most memorable service to military medicine, and his most enduring legacy, was the introductory use of ligatures to tie off blood vessels leading to damaged or missing limbs. This new surgical innovation not only led to less (and in many cases what was usually fatal) blood loss, but directly to the more effective and life-saving use of amputations to deal with the ever-increasing numbers of shattered and useless limbs resulting from both the increasing use of the arquebus and ever more effective and efficient cannons.

What was not lost in all this was the fact that Paré was adored by the army as well as esteemed by successive French kings, while at the same time all of his innovations were not only challenged, but opposed by the medical establishment and the faculties of the medical academic centers of Europe. It may be true that in medicine, as in most sciences, the advances proceed more funeral-by-funeral than idea-by-idea.

Amazingly, much of the same antagonism and arguments used against Paré's innovations are now occurring among physicians and surgeons regarding the best treatments for our newest battlefield injuries—blast injuries to the body and the brain—that so conflicted and confounded the contemporaries of Paré when first faced with gunshot wounds.

Once again, the battlefield has yielded up medical questions whose solutions will eventually affect all of us, whether or not we are deployed and whether or not we ever pick up a weapon or fire a machine gun. The concentrated suffering and deaths on battlefields have always, though at a terrible price, been the workshops for better medical and surgical care.

The Second World War gave us, and the world, plasma, nutritionally effective K-rations, and the wide use of the sulfa and penicillin antibiotics that had been discovered in the late 1930s. The Vietnam War gave us, and the world, methods of rapid evacuations of the wounded and the ability to keep victims alive during that golden hour after an injury when ultimate survival still exists. All this commitment of effort, steadfastness of purpose, and splendid behavior in the face of unbelievable danger, is a quintessential American thing. Nobody really told anyone to do it. It was done just because it was a better and right way to do things and because the need was there. So we did it.

There has always been an implicit sense of practicality to Americans. It was something Alexis de Tocqueville noted in his travels through the United States in the early Nineteenth Century and remains today a part of our national character. Americans will always do what works, whatever the sacrifice.

In World War II, Korea, and Vietnam, it led to a bravery and self-sacrifice that became as commonplace as it was scary. The medics in Vietnam did what they did without complaint, because they understood that minutes did matter and keeping soldiers alive long enough for the choppers to get in did work.

At a time when dissent was becoming a way of life and rebellion was growing into an attitude, the continuing courage and self-denial of the medics was an extraordinary thing to witness. Even within an army being abandoned at the very edge of empire, the medics successfully struggled to keep their own alive.

Looked at objectively, what the medics did in Vietnam was not that sophisticated. No one expected the medics to devise a comprehensive treatment plan or make any detailed medical assessments. They were not expected to do brain surgery or put in an arterial line. They were doing ambulance medicine: pack the wounds, stop the bleeding, give fluids, maintain blood pressures, try to keep the heart going and keep everyone breathing until the med-evac choppers flew in.

Courage, determination, sacrifice, and bravery made it all work, but the lynch pin both emotionally and operationally of U.S. combat medicine in 'Nam was the anticipation of both a rapid and a timely evacuation of the wounded. For the next twenty-five years, that was the universal standard of battlefield medical care. There was no thought of changing procedures, and certainly no effort to change the training of combat medics.

All of that ended on the afternoon of October 3, 1993, when a search-and-rescue team rappelled down from a hovering helicopter into the streets of Mogadishu, Somalia. What should have been no more than a rescue mission protecting the distribution of foodstuffs by the United Nations to refugees of the Somali civil war, had morphed into a search-and-destroy mission to capture or kill one of Somalia's major warlords.

The "can-do" attitude of the military had merged with the hubris of our government, sending an undermanned unit—with a lack of armor and fire support—to take on the Somalis in their own city, in the worst of all possible combat zones: the narrow streets and alleys of a crowded urban center.

Those U.S. Army Rangers and Special Forces troopers who rope-dropped into Mogadishu quickly found themselves under a siege that would continue uninterrupted for three days, becoming the longest and deadliest firefight involving an American combat unit since the Vietnam War. The battle fought in those narrow streets and alleys changed everything in both the theory and practice of U.S. combat medicine.

The minute-by-minute specifics of the battle were described by the journalist, Mark Bowden, in his *Blackhawk Down*. During what was really a seventy-two-hour gunfight, eighteen Rangers and Special Forces troopers were killed, two helicopters were shot down—showing once again the dangers of using vulnerable helicopters in the narrowed spaces of an urban landscape—and over a hundred of the 170 U.S. soldiers involved in the battle were wounded. Thousands of Somalis were killed. What had begun as a simple search-and-arrest operation quickly became a desperate fight for survival.

The medics who, along with the Rangers, rappelled down to the first crash site, came under intense fire the moment they hit the ground. Several members of the rescue team were hit while the medics, a number wounded themselves, had to deal with more and more casualties as the battle continued.

True, the original mission had nothing to do with combat but rather with the distribution of humanitarian aid. But there was "mission-creep" and the mission quickly morphed into one of capturing a Somalia warlord—becoming a combat mission that was attempted without tanks, armored personnel carriers, or up-armored Humvees. It was simply forgotten or ignored that during actual combat armored units are usually necessary for long-term survival.

Apparently, neither the Department of Defense nor the Joint Chiefs of Staff thought there would be any prolonged battles, or that tanks and armored personnel carriers would be necessary. The siege of the U.S. troops was lifted only after the American command was able to borrow armored personnel carriers from Pakistani units on the other side of the city.

Through that first afternoon and night of the siege, the entire next day and night, and most of the rest of the next day, the medics had no choice but to care for the increasing numbers of wounded on their own. Additional choppers could not get in to reinforce the surrounded troops and bring in more ammunition and medical supplies, nor could the medics get the casualties out.

In the words of one of the medics, "I gave IV fluids to people who had uncomplicated gunshot wounds in the arms and legs. They were fine, but I wasted time starting IVs and I wasted fluids and then when I had someone with a pretty significant vascular injury, I was out of fluids. What we did was stupid."

There is a maxim in the military that "you fight the way you train." What happened in Somalia was not stupid as much as out-of-date. Apparently while no one had been looking, the kind of wars we had begun to fight had changed. Our government and the Pentagon had sent our troops and medics into Somalia having been trained for the past.

In the setting of urban warfare, where choppers are at even greater risk than ground troops, the medical practices that had begun in World War II, and were fine-tuned in Vietnam— maintaining airways, stopping bleeding, giving intravenous fluids to maintain vascular volumes, and blood pressures, all focused on the goal of a rapid and effective medical evacuation—suddenly proved worthless. Within hours of rope-dropping into the streets of Mogadishu, the medics had used up all their IVs, all their plasma, all their tourniquets, and all their morphine, leaving nothing for the wounded they could not get out and nothing for the increasing numbers of new casualties coming in. It was not the training that had lost its effectiveness; it was the battlefield that had changed. Mogadishu was clearly the tipping point, the final wake-up call, forcing the military to abandon the last of its practices from Vietnam: the care of its wounded.

The 1991 Persian Gulf War never really tested the established medical doctrine of stabilization of casualties, followed by rapid chopper evacuations. There was no need. That war was fought out in the open, with half a million troops spread through five heavy divisions and dozens of armored regiments with complete battlefield and air superiority. As then Chairman of the Joint Chiefs of Staff, General Colin Powell, explained at the first press conference after the start of the war, the focus was to be on, "Finding Saddam's army, fixing them in place and killing them." The war lasted only 100 hours, with less than 300 deaths and a large percentage of those killed the results of friendly fire. Overwhelming military force proved the effectiveness of what was called the Powell-Weinberger Military Doctrine, named for both Colin Powell and Secretary of Defense Casper Weinberger, that basically stated: no war without putting in place adequate resources to accomplish the reason for going to war.

But then came Mogadishu in 1993 and Kosovo in 1999 and half a dozen other military interventions. The rules and decisions on committing our armed forces were also changing. To achieve its international goals, our government was becoming more predisposed toward military options than the use of diplomacy. U.S. presidents were growing increasingly more willing to send troops into all kinds of circumstances in every corner of the world, using smaller and more agile units to fight in ever more distant and difficult terrains. The majority of these actions were behind enemy lines or along very long and sparsely defended supply routes.

There was now little chance of the wounded being medevaced in a timely fashion. Medics would clearly have to learn a new trade. They would have to be able to keep casualties alive, without the possibility of evacuation, for up to seventy-two hours. A study by military physicians analyzing every serious injury and death that had occurred in Mogadishu following the battle documented what had gone wrong, along with what procedures and policies might have unwittingly led to all deaths.

The study showed that several of the casualties had bled to death from wounds where direct pressure to stop the bleeding could not be applied, such as wounds to the head and neck as well as the chest, abdomen, and groin. Many of the new recommendations were already in place within the military, but Somalia clearly accelerated the process. It was time to change from triage to intensive care.

The training period for the Combat Medical Specialty was increased from ten to sixteen weeks. The former 91B Military Occupational Specialty of Combat Medic was reclassified 91W as "Health Care Specialist." All trainees were required to pass the civilian Emergency Medical Technician (EMT) test.

The additional weeks of training were devoted to developing the core skills necessary to keep the severely wounded alive where they were hit, with little chance for immediate evacuation. No more "patch 'em up and send them off." This was to be big-time medicine, the city trauma unit brought to the battlefield.

The training added hands-on courses using high-tech patient simulators that could accurately mimic battlefield injuries, from respiratory failure to penetrating head wounds and transected spinal cords—in real time and under combat conditions. A "bleeding lab" set up to duplicate any number of hemorrhaging wounds became part of the program. The models used in the training actually would "bleed to death" if the blood loss was not stopped. The simulations are so real that the dummies really do "suffocate" if the chest tubes are not correctly placed or a tracheotomy performed within the required three minutes.

The military also incorporated the most recent and relevant advances in trauma surgery into the medical training. They moved to the evolving intensive-care treatment of hypotensive resuscitation, where blood, plasma, or IV fluids are given only in minimal amounts solely to keep the heart pumping, rather than the old World War II, Korean, and Vietnam method of resuscitation, where blood pressures were maintained at normal or elevated levels.

In a tragic and ironic way, these new medical and surgical procedures were found to work better for combat casualties than for civilian gunshot wounds, train, motorcycle, or car accidents. Combat troopers are basically healthy young men and women up until the time they are hit. In these patients, unlike civilian injuries where the patients might be older, likely out of shape, overweight with high blood pressure and diabetes, and often on three to five medications, you can sacrifice a little blood pressure to keep the life-saving blood clots from "popping loose" when blood pressures are raised too quickly or kept above normal levels for too long a time. Hypotensive resuscitation allows early clots to stay in place and new clots to form. It is always the bleeding that kills you on the battlefield.

But hypotensive blood and fluid replacement have an additional value. The large, cumbersome bottles and bags of plasma and IV fluids needed under the old techniques have been replaced by high-tech starch concentrate solutions, allowing medics to haul around fewer medical supplies while being able to care for more casualties over longer periods of time. Better-designed tourniquets, along with the hemostatic embedded dressings and stents, have also been introduced for better local hemorrhage control.

Medics are also taught a technique for evaluating a patient's blood volume status that goes back to Hippocrates: by first looking at the patient, talking to them to establish their degree of consciousness, and taking a pulse. Patients in impending shock from blood loss experience mental confusion, while it is easy and immediate to characterize a pulse as "absent," "weak," or "normal." Those with absent or weak pulses are given whole blood as quickly as possible. It is on such simple yet sophisticated assessments that modern life-saving decisions are made.

An early analysis of "potentially survivable" wounds in soldiers and marines in Iraq who died after reaching a hospital showed that over 80 percent died because of ongoing hemorrhage, 70 percent from continued or recurrent bleeding from what the military calls "non-tourniquetable" wound sites. A soldier or marine with a torn pelvic artery or a severed femoral artery that is too high up in the thigh to be clamped, or if the wound suddenly begins to re-bleed, will die within minutes.

With development and the use of what is called "combat gauze," a surgical pack that contains a powder that causes clotting simply by being put into a wound, has proved effective in stopping bleeding from wounds that cannot be stopped with a tourniquet. There is a new medication called Nova 7, used by neurosurgeons to stop bleeding within the brain during surgical procedures. It is used when surgeons cannot tie off any major blood vessels without damaging the healthy parts of the brain needing an adequate blood supply to remain healthy and function properly. Nova 7, costing over a 1,000 dollars a gram, is a medication that will clot off bleeding blood vessels. It is given IV and is now being carried by medics. The problem with the use of any clotting medication is that the medication will also clot off undamaged and healthy vessels, a problem in the elderly and those whose clotting systems are already stressed or damaged. But our troops are basically young and healthy and can handle the medication without complications. The use of Nova 7 right there on the battlefield is a quantum leap in saving lives.

But now, the almost universal use of whole blood rather than the IV fluids and plasma used in World War II, Korea, and Vietnam to treat shock has made the greatest difference between our wounded living or dying.

Blood is basically a mixture of 45 percent circulating red blood cells that carry oxygen to all the organs of the body and 55 percent plasma that contains water, salts, sugars, fats, hormones, and the dozen circulating proteins that make up the body's clotting factors. It is these clotting factors, working together in a complicated biochemical way, that causes blood to clot. Patients with hemophilia have a genetic absence of one of these factors, given the innocuous name of Factor 8, that can not only cause significant internal bleeding but can lead to the patient bleeding to death even from minor cuts or injuries, including tooth extractions. The problem is that any trauma patient will, if injured enough, consume their own circulating clotting factors and continue to bleed or re-bleed as these factors are not replaced. Unfortunately, if transfusions following a traumatic injury are made up mostly of oxygen-carrying red cells and stored plasma or IV fluids alone, simple bleeding can become a re-bleed that quickly cascades into a fatal hemorrhage. What works to keep soldiers and marines alive, even after massive traumatic injuries, is the use of whole blood or the infusions of the individual clotting factor proteins in a timely fashion. And that is what happens today in both Iraq and Afghanistan. Whole blood's magical powers to save our newest trauma victims are now clearly understood and its use along with the other battlefield techniques of evaluation and wound treatments has made it more difficult to die than in any of our other wars at any other time in our country's history.

In addition, today's medics are taught to give antibiotics earlier and in much larger dosages than in the past. The deeper and more extensive the wounds, and that is mostly the case today in Afghanistan, the greater the risk of immediate or later infections. Medics also have begun to use the latest non-opioid painkillers that, unlike morphine, Demerol and oral codeine, do not depress respiration. Dying simply doesn't happen as frequently as it has in the past. There is a new "normal" out there on our battlefields and it is that new normal that we are all going to have to deal with, as well as understand.

There is little doubt that today's medics can keep casualties alive for days, until that chopper or overland relief finally arrives, and that the physicians, surgeons, and nurses all along the evac chain can now manage to hold off death itself.

But unfortunately our wars have clearly changed on us. There is no doubt that despite the pronouncements of "Mission Accomplished" the war in Iraq did not end with the defeat of Saddam's army. The war turned into an insurgency and the combatants, aware of the well-publicized overwhelming firepower of the U.S. military, gave up direct military confrontations. They stepped up their use of IEDs, choosing support troops and supply convoys rather than the more heavily-armed, protected, and aggressive combat units.

When our military added more armor to the units moving through hostile areas, the insurgents switched to the more powerful car and roadside bombs, increasing the power and blast radius of their IEDs. Unlike all our other wars, today's injuries, rather than coming from ahead and above, are coming from behind, below, and from the sides.

Regular Army combat units and National Guard and Reserve troops started losing arms and legs and suffering head injuries at unexpected and unanticipated rates. Overwhelmed by the increasing numbers of mangled limbs, eye injuries, penetrating head wounds, and closed head trauma, the upgraded medical training following Mogadishu began to lose its edge for the medical personnel.

Yet, despite the severity and grievousness of the new wounds, death rates have not increased. The explosive charges that now blow off arms and legs and lead to traumatic brain injuries (TBIs), would, in Vietnam, have killed those troops right there where the blasts occurred. The penetrating chest wounds, ruptured aortas, shattered livers and spleens, transected spinal cords and fractured kidneys, along with the collapsed lungs and the massive internal hemorrhages that had always gone along with severe extremity wounds and head injuries, had usually proved uniformly and quickly fatal. Those casualties with mangled or lost limbs, and those with brain and spinal cord injuries, rarely made it alive to the chopper, much less the nearest surgical or evac hospital. That is simply no longer the case.

Those military surgeons familiar with Vietnam spoke with amazement early in the war in Iraq, when they first removed the body armor from the newest med-evacs and could not find a scratch from chin to groin. Yet these casualties had arms and legs that were mangled along with head injuries that were horrific. But none of them bled to death. The body armor had spared the wounded shattered organs, and the unstoppable internal bleeding that uniformly led to a rapid, devastating, unstoppable blood loss followed quickly by death. You can live with half your brain gone as long as the deep centers keep you breathing and your intact heart remains pumping. And you can live if a limb is blown off and a tourniquet or vascular clamp is quickly placed to stop the bleeding.

As Clausewitz pointed out in his book, *On War* coining the memorable and accurate phrase "the Fog of War," nothing in war is ever as simple or as straightforward as it first appears. And that applies to our troops surviving the terrible wounds of our present wars.

Survival is not solely the result of better body armor protecting the vital organs and major blood vessels in the chest and upper abdomen, nor is it the more effective and quick use of tourniquets, or the improved medical training for medics. Casualties survived because the whole military medical system has itself become both more mobile and more agile.

These new wars, under the current doctrine of "Faster, Lighter, Quicker," places a limited number of boots—a so-called "light footprint," on the ground. The need for widely dispersed units shuffling from border to border and town to town, along with the increasing severity of the peripheral body wounds, demanded a more sophisticated medical support that moved along with the different units. There was a need for an evacuation system that went beyond the post-Mogadishu "keep them alive for seventy-two hours" approach.

Out of both common sense as well as the need to support a faster and lighter military, the Army devised and instituted a new concept of frontline battlefield medical care: The Forward Surgical Teams, or FSTs.

These teams are in essence upgrades of the old MASH (Mobile Army Surgical Hospital) units of the Korean War era, only smaller and more nimble and in a strange way better equipped for their one specific task: survival. The typical team consists of fewer than twenty medical personnel: three general surgeons, one orthopedic surgeon, two nurse anesthetists, three nurses, and a few medics. Each FST travels in six Humvees. The transport vehicles carry three RATs (Rapid Assembly Tents) that can be set up in less than sixty minutes and attached to each other to form a 900-foot long surgical facility.

FSTs are decidedly lean affairs. There is no high-tech radiographic equipment. Surgeons detect fractures by feel, but there are operating tables, ultrasonic equipment, modern anesthesia packs, and high-tech ventilators.

These mobile units are not based on the major trauma centers that led to the EMT training of combat medics. The FSTs aim only for damage control. There is no effort at definitive repair. The surgeons seek to limit all operations to less than two hours, preferably to less than an hour. Abdomens are left open, bowels left unattached or connected to large drains, fractured livers simply packed to control bleeding, dirty wounds washed out, torn and useless bones and tissues quickly removed.

There are also the rapid evacuations back to the States. In Vietnam, the average time from the battlefield to the States was forty-five days; the average time now from Mosul or Nasharia to the hospital at Landstuhl, Germany is less than eighteen hours, and then on to Walter Reed or Bethesda Naval Hospital in the States within the next three days.

More importantly, even the number of those who do not survive after they reach a major surgical facility has decreased. But in military support hospitals in Iraq and Afghanistan, or in the neurosurgical ward at Landstuhl Regional Medical Center, the poly-trauma unit at Walter Reed or the orthopedic wards at Bethesda Naval Hospital, along with the Rehab and PTSD clinics in the Veteran Administration's hospitals, survival no longer gives the entire picture of our newest wars, nor what have become the real and substantial risks that the majority of our wounded soldiers and marines actually do face.

Despite what you may have read about the dangers facing our troops fighting in Iraq and now in ever larger numbers in Afghanistan, the real truth is much closer to the comments of a nurse at the Twenty-fourth Combat Support Hospital in Baghdad:

We're saving more people who shouldn't be saved. We're saving the really severely injured, legs gone, eyes blinded, deaf, parts of brains destroyed. You may get home, but you wouldn't be the same as when you left.

And those that the nurse talks about now number into the tens of thousands.

Behind every fatality in Iraq and now Afghanistan there lies a hidden cost that few in the military seem to understand and even fewer among Washington's policy makers seem to have fully grasped. Certainly the media, as well as political pundits, have refused to see the obvious.

Since September 2001, the Air Force's Air Mobility Command, using the C-17 military transport aircraft that form the air ambulances that fly the wounded from Iraq and Afghanistan back to the Continental United States, landing mainly out of sight at restricted air bases, have flown some 30,000 aero-medical evacuation missions transporting over 150,000 patients. These evacuation flights have been cobbled together from various National Guard and Air Force Reserve units. Some of these squadrons have been routinely and constantly deployed, some a dozen or so times, six months of the year. This rapid evacuation back to the United States is part of the new approach of military medicine. As one of the flight surgeons explained:

"We've adopted an entirely different vision of combat medical care than we had back in Vietnam. During that era, the military

built huge hospitals in combat theaters, as close to the battlefield as practical to quickly care for the wounded. Now we are fighting multiple wars with very dispersed and fluid front lines, which means we don't have the luxury of having huge hospitals near the action. So the psychology of medical care has changed to rapidly stabilizing the patients on the ground and then flying them back to the United States to receive definitive care as quickly as possible ... "

But with all this, not everyone survives. Even with the newest technology, the effort and the speed, not everyone makes it. Some become brain dead during the first part of the flights home. More than one set of parents waiting in Germany to meet their sons and daughters have flown back to the States with the bodies, many to donate the soldier's organs. Some of the docs and nurses working these flights have a more focused and more realistic view of their work than the rest of us:

We get these boys home so they can either get better, or we keep them alive long enough for their families to say goodbye.

James Kitfield, the Pentagon correspondent for the *National Journal* who made such a flight back to the States aptly wrote for the May 2010 issue of the *Journal:*

No matter how one feels about the conflicts in Iraq and Afghanistan, every American could benefit from spending time in the company of the wars' wounded and maimed. Watching these young men and women clinging to life, at the mercy of machines that count their every breath and heart beat ... a witness confronts an inescapable thought.

The same thought surely occurred to President Obama when he traveled last October to the tarmac at Dover Air Force Base in Delaware to meet the flag-draped caskets of fallen service members returning from Afghanistan in the middle of the night: This had better be worth it.

Indeed.

8.

Teleconferencing / More Than Six Degrees of Separation

In a very real way every generation deserves the wounds they get ...

—military surgeon, 2010

There is a new normal in medicine today and that new normal has worked its way into military medicine and definitely has become the norm for battlefield care. It is no longer expertise in medicine or surgery that is expected, that much, for better or worse, is simply assumed. It is technology. X-rays once read exclusively on the view boxes of radiology departments in every hospital in America were always connected to a patient as well as a name and possible diagnosis. But when these images became digitalized as data points and could be sent through phone lines and satellite connections anywhere in the world at almost the speed of light, the patient was lost. It is true that today many of the X-rays, flat plates of the abdomen, CT scans, and MRIs taken at night in your hospital are sent to India to be read, the results texted back within minutes, eliminating the need and the expense of the hospital to have to pay for a radiologist on call twenty-four hours a day, seven days a week.

The use of the newly-developed robotic surgery allows surgeons in New York, using a "slave machine," to operate in real time on a patient in an operating room in Iowa. In reality, you no longer need to have a physician physically present to see or even examine a patient. A moveable robot with its own camera as a videocam, a motorized tread connected to a two-way microphone, and voice-box operated with a joy stick by an expert in, say neurology, at some remote location, can with the help of a trained surrogate, ask the important neurological questions and actually perform a credible physical examination.

It used to be that you knew the physicians who diagnosed and took care of your heart attack or the surgeon who did your coronary by-pass. Now the cardiologist who puts in the stent to unplug your coronary artery an hour after you have your chest pain is someone you never saw before, someone you never knew, and someone who most likely you will never see again. It is the same with the gastroenterologist who does your colonoscopy, and after removing the polyp in your colon tells you that you will need another colonoscopy in five years even as he leaves the examination room. The new paradigm of medicine lies in the technology and it is only to be expected that the benefits and the downside of this kind of anonymous medical and surgical care has been brought to the battlefield. And why not? It works.

Medicine is always easier when it is only the technical aspects that are in play. In referral hospitals across the country over 80 percent of all pacemakers are put into patients well over eighty-five years of age. If you are only discussing the functions of the heart and not the whole patient, then these numbers might make sense. What no one knows, because it is not asked, is how many of these patients over eighty-five have dementia or other disabling and untreatable chronic conditions. The cardiologist simply becomes the technician, or the more accepted term "provider." And apparently they do provide.

Once a week, the physicians, nurses, and surgeons at all the combat hospitals in Afghanistan, in Europe, and in the United States, linked by telephones and videocams, meet over a secure internet connection to discuss those patients wounded during the preceding week. It is all business, with experts in all the fields of medicine and surgery from orthopedics to neurosurgery to infectious diseases, as well as occupational therapists, medical and surgical nurses and nurse practitioners taking part, even if they have never talked to each other before and are in rooms more then 16,000 miles apart. The focus is only on the injuries and not the patient. There is no time for ethics or moral decisions here. There are little or no personal conversations. The majority of physicians and surgeons in the conferences have never met one another. Indeed, the participants are not referred to by name since no one really knows anyone else and so the discussions are called out by location, "Ballad," "Kandahar," "Landstuhl," "Fort Sam Houston," "Walter Reed."

These last years of changing wounds in Iraq, and now throughout Afghanistan, have taken battlefield medicine well past rapid med-evacs and even Forward Surgical Teams. The Mash Unit and even the Evac hospitals with wounded staying hours and hours, if not days or weeks, are things of the past. There is no need now for lengthy hospitalizations at any one facility along the evac chain. There is certainly no longer the need for a Camp Zama in some distant country, nor is there time for long individual discussions or thoughtful contemplative postures. Today, in civilian hospitals and certainly military hospitals, with the fragmentation of medicine itself into its different specialties, there is the need for an abundance of different medical and surgical personnel to take care of the multiple needs of soldiers and marines who are blown up while, at the same time, being exposed to enormous shock waves of these IED blasts. Few if any military physicians will see the wounded longer than a few hours or a few days, before the patients are moved on to what has become trans-continental care, with survival being the single goal.

The truth is that with the new kinds of battlefield injuries, this is precisely the kind of care that is needed because it is efficient, technically sound, and, more importantly, it can now be done. With the new understanding of wounds, injuries, and the new technologies, and the fact that the wounded are usually young and fit, there is no one to "hang the crepe" unless the shroud is ready. After all, this isn't cancer or strokes, these are accidents—immediate and complicated, but still accidents, and that is precisely how they are viewed and how they are treated.

All of this, taken together, is called "Damage Control Surgery" which began in Iraq but is being perfected, out of necessity, in Afghanistan. The point, obvious to everyone involved with military medicine and those on the weekly telecommunication calls, is that because of the new type of hyper-technical divided expert care, the vast majority of these patients are not what they had always been in every one of our other wars, dead within hours, if not days, of being hit. It is hard to ignore the virtue in all that.

The fact that today's wounds are now attended to in stages is not genius but the fact that years of experience within civil trauma centers has shown that the more severe and complicated trauma patients survive if their various injuries are treated incrementally in a well-organized step-wise fashion. And that is exactly the types of wounds we are getting in Afghanistan and in ever increasing numbers.

As one of the Navy surgeons deployed to Kandahar Air Field recently explained:

"Twenty years ago, if you left the operating room without fixing everything, you weren't a good surgeon. We don't believe that anymore."

But the reason for no longer practicing that kind of trauma surgery is because our troops are no longer being shot at; they are being blown up. They suffer from multiple wounds, terrible and contaminated by projectiles and the dirt and dust set into motion by the explosions. Unlike simple bullet wounds that can be dealt with quickly and usually with one surgery, these wounds, because of their various body locations and differing severities, along with the multiple types of contamination, have to be treated by stages with as little done at each surgery as possible.

This type of limited surgery is a medical requirement because, initially, no one knows or can determine with any accuracy the exact extent of the wounds. The nature of blast injuries is such that the extent of the injuries only becomes obvious over time. Often it is one surgery per hospital at a time, and the patient is passed on down the line to the next and more sophisticated group of surgeons and physicians, until finally reaching one of the giant medical centers in the States.

The term Improvised Explosive Device or IED is clearly a misnomer. There is nothing improvised about these blasts and what are now being called "Dismounted IED Injuries" to designate wounds caused by a bomb that injures a soldier or marine outside of a vehicle. These weapons blowing up soldiers, outside or under or beside a vehicle, explode with deadly force resulting in such widespread and extensive injuries that no one surgery can fix all the injuries, much less the patient, at any one time or with any one procedure.

IEDs break bones and blow off limbs and drive dirt deep into the opened wounds while the shock waves kill cells and damage tissues. It may take hours or even days to become evident. In the new damage-control surgery, these wounds are washed out, the obvious dead tissue removed often under repeated anesthesia, the increasingly dead tissues removed bit by bit even if the removals necessitate ever wider and more extensive surgeries, and repeated amputations over days or weeks.

It is the same with abdominal wounds. With any penetrating chest or abdomen wound, the chests and abdomens of these kids are explored and re-explored, the surgeons looking for additional organ damage and any newly leaking blood vessels or veins that might have been missed during previous explorations and surgeries. It is here that the advances of vascular surgery, including the placement of patches and grafts developed to treat the wounds of Vietnam, become so important.

In Afghanistan the pelvic blast injuries are particularly massive and difficult to treat. It is the common in-between-the-leg blasts set off by soldiers on patrol that routinely take off both legs as well as the genitals while causing massive internal injuries to the bladder, colon, and pelvic bones. New wars—new weapons—new injuries—new treatments and procedures—a new kind of suffering.

The new techniques of battlefield medicine have become one long and desperate surgery that may go on for weeks and months and even years. Maybe those who sent our troops into Iraq and Afghanistan, and keep sending them there, should have known all this would happen. They could argue they didn't know and couldn't have known. But they know now.

It is probably true that none of these kids would, with similar injuries, survive out in the civilian world, or that they could have been saved in either Iraq or Afghanistan just five years ago. But that isn't the issue. It is almost counter-intuitive, but as a physician or surgeon it is always a bit easier, if that is the word for it, to give up on a desperately ill or damaged patient if you know them and if you know the family, and have a sense of what survival will actually mean in the long term to both the patient and their loved ones.

When you talk to military surgeons about what they do, they will tell you that they don't feel their efforts are futile even in the face of treating a 90 percent burn victim, or a patient with all four limbs amputated, or those who need a respirator to breathe. But this new type of "Damage Control Surgery" is a kind of shift work where everyone does their own thing and the big picture is lost in the effort, or left up to someone else down the line to deal with, which in the final analysis will be the family. Today's battlefield physicians save lives. It is what they do because they can do it. But if you push them, they admit that they try not to withdraw care in the combat theater, but then admit that, every now and then, they will stop all cares. But that is usually with the severe head injuries where the wounded would likely die in transport. Then they make sure that those soldiers die where they are, with other troops by the bedside. "It just affords them that last little bit of dignity." And when they admit that much, their voices usually crack and their eyes fill with tears—

9.

ALL THE TOMS / IRAQ / 2004

We have a volunteer army and have had one since the late 1970s. There is no draft. Yet of all the three services, the Marines, except for Vietnam, have never needed one. Organized in 1775 to fight on both sea and land before the founding of the Republic, the Marines have always been a volunteer force. It was only the enormous casualties of the early years of the Vietnam War, fought in a country of mountains and jungles, a landscape set up for war, that forced sergeants in induction centers across the country, beginning in early 1968, to walk down the lines of newly arrived draftees tapping each third young man on the shoulder as an unceremonious induction into the Marines.

Those young men knew, if they knew nothing else, it might well be that fateful tap. Marines were being killed platoon by platoon in the elephant grass of the Central Highlands and along the Laotian border. A joke had begun going around the Marine Corps early in the Vietnam War that the reason there were so few captains in charge of companies was that they had all been killed as second lieutenants. Lieutenants, captains, majors, and non-commissioned officers were being killed and wounded alongside enlisted personnel in numbers that, at times, made filling all the empty slots difficult, if not impossible.

When units of the First Air Cav replaced the Marines following the three-month siege of Khe Sanh—a Marine outpost in

Northern Quang Tri Province—in late 1967, the Cav troopers were astonished to find that the Marines—despite the hourly mortar and rocket attacks, had never dug in and were walking around the hill tops of the siege area in flack vests and helmets. The officers of the First Cav asked the Marine officers why they hadn't built more defensive positions. The official, as well as unofficial, answer was " You can't kill 'em if you're in a bunker."

Being drafted to go to 'Nam was one thing, being sent as a marine was quite another. Karl Marlente captures it perfectly in his novel *Matterhorn*. In the late 1960s and early 70s you didn't have to read a book about Vietnam to understand what was happening. Everyone in America, unlike today, knew about their war. They knew that their country had sent over half a million troops to make the fight. They knew about Khe Sanh and the Tet Offensive and they knew about the casualties. Our battles, as well as the number of deaths and casualties, were constantly on the evening news and written about daily in the newspapers.

We now have a military, rather than a country, at war and we have a volunteer army and a constantly deployed National Guard rather than a draft to supply our military with enough troops to make a fight. But those who still chose to go into the Marines, like the marines themselves, haven't changed. They are still a bit different from the rest of the military and the rest of us.

The gangs in East Los Angeles, if not the rest of us, understand that much about our wars, as well the dangers faced by our marines. The LA police will tell you that it is a well-understood fact that you cannot get out of these gangs once you become a member. Being in a gang is a lifetime commitment, unless you go into the Marines. If you finish the four-year commitment and get safely back home you can decide if you want to go back into the gang or simply walk away. It is an agreement of sorts that indeed, the Marines are different. The gangs understand that there are no short cuts where survival is due either to luck or the ability to kill someone before they kill you. In either case, you deserve admiration and at the very minimum, respect. That clearly seems to be something missing from the rest of the country, or at least most of it. But not all—

There are still other volunteers. It doesn't happen all that often. But when it does happen, it usually happens like this. A bright eighteen-year-old kid decides that college is not for him and that a job flipping hamburgers at McDonald's or Burger King is not all that appealing. He asks around and somehow finds out that the Marines have a deferred enlistment program available at the end of the senior year of high school that allows recruits their choice of any of the three Military Occupational Specialties: Artillery, Tanks, or Low Level Anti-aircraft. Always interested in cars and trucks, and realizing the advantage of choosing the type of duty he wants, or at least fancies, the eighteen-year-old chooses to be a tanker and decides to enlist at the beginning of his senior year. Whatever else happens, at least he will not have to walk into battle.

The parents are not happy and take their son aside to caution him that this should not be a frivolous or casual decision and that there are real, grown-up consequences to joining the military, including being killed or being wounded. But "Tom" will have none of it, insisting that he will be careful. The parents, understanding that their child is a bit lost, and that the military is better than sitting around not really doing anything, reluctantly agree. The military will give him the chance to grow up. Besides, what other options are there? For many if not most, the volunteer Army or Marines is as much a way out, as it is a way up.

You don't need much to sign up, just be free of drugs, pass a normal physical examination, and not have a criminal record. The Marines will take care of the rest. And so, with his parents unwilling, but unable to stop or dissuade him, Tom is in the Marines a month after high school graduation.

Two weeks later, he is on his way to thirteen weeks of basic training. He is strangely pleased and oddly comforted that basic training in the Marines is the longest and most demanding of all the armed forces. He even appreciates that the Marines separate the female from the male recruits during basic training. It wasn't sexism, he simply viewed the women as probably slowing the rest of them down.

And there was talk from the very beginning of basic about the "Crucible," the three days of hell to get through at the end of basic that would not only separate the men from the boys, but the winners from the losers. Tom might be young, but he is no fool. He knew he'd make it through the Crucible. He understood that if you wanted to be the best, you had to know how to be the best. And he was willing to learn.

Tom never wavered once, not even during the Crucible, which he found to be the most difficult thing, physically and mentally, he'd ever done in his life. Pushed to the limit while testing his own perseverance and teamwork, he was amazed that he'd actually gotten through the three days without giving up or quitting. It was heady stuff. The core values of being a Marine were no longer what had been presented that first day of basic—Duty, Honor, Country—but had morphed into Commitment, Courage, and Responsibility, and simply deciding not to fail. And he had done it without failing and without complaining. He finally understood what someone told him that a climber had said about why he'd wanted to climb Everest, "Because It Is There." That is what becomes so life changing, at eighteen or at sixty-five.

After basic training, Tom went to four weeks of MCT (Marine Combat Training). In the Army, it's called Advanced Infantry Training, but for the Marines, it is simply something everyone does.

MCT was a month of weapons firing and weapons management. Tom learned how to use all the individual and crew-served weapons in the Marine arsenal. There was little joking around now, and fewer attempts at humor. Weapons are a serious business. Everyone understood that this was no longer training, but potentially life and death.

Following MCT, Tom went on to two and a half months of tank school at Fort Knox, where he learned machinery, maintenance, and some gunnery. On the second day out on the tank course, he knew he'd made the right choice.

The M1A1 battle tank had a 120-millimeter smooth bore cannon. The British Challenger 2 Main Battle Tank, used by

NATO forces in Southern Iraq, has a 120-millimeter rifled barrel. But the rounds from the M1A1 have a higher muzzle velocity than the British cannon, leaving the gun at more than 3,200 feet per second, which meant better accuracy than the Challenger 2 up to and beyond 3,000 yards. There was simply no contest with the Russian tanks.

The M1A1 weighed seventy tons and, with its gas turbine engine, could go through or over anything at fifty miles an hour. Whatever else anyone might think of U.S. armor, he'd definitely be the biggest kid on the block.

There was more training, more honing of skills, along with a better understanding of what it was to be a Marine and then what it was to be a Marine at war. Tom liked it all. He liked the camaraderie. He liked the effort and being a part of something bigger than himself. He liked the sense of responsibility and even of honor. He even liked the crusty old sergeants who never married because the Corps had never issued them a wife.

Following tank school, Tom became a member of Alpha Company, First Tank Battalion, First Marine Division. Six months after the fall of Baghdad in April 2003, he arrived with Alpha Company, First Battalion to become part of a regimental combat team designated RCT 2.

The Marines, despite the pronouncements coming out of Washington that the war had been won, understood that the war had simply changed. It did not take a military genius to understand that when you have more casualties in supply units than in regular front line troops, you don't have enough grunts on the ground to make the fight, much less to guard your supply routes, and definitely not enough troops to hold the peace. More than one Marine combat unit had noticed in their run up from Nasiriya to Baghdad at the beginning of the war that, as they pulled out of a town, they could hear increasing firing behind them, but didn't have enough troops to go back and see what was going on. The war was quickly transforming itself into an insurgency even as those in Washington were landing on aircraft carriers under the banner of "Mission Accomplished."

The Marine Command distributed their tanks among the combat platoons, putting the tanks up front with the troops on the ground, rumbling through the streets of Iraq's towns and villages, inching forward side by side with the grunts as they moved past roadblocks and swept through towns and villages, supplying both covering fire power to the ground units and, when necessary, immediate backup.

The tactics and rules of engagement for an RCT (Regimental Combat Team) are as simple as they are straightforward. Ground units move forward with their tanks for cover. The tanks, with their enormous weight and firepower, keep pace with the grunts. It is an intimate and immediate kind of warfare, a dance that Tom learned to admire and then appreciate, even though it was a dance that left little room for error and absolutely none for a mistake. Marines have never been nation builders, nor are they promoters of democracy. They put themselves in harm's way to kill people and break things and an RTC is an effective machine to do just that.

And that is what happened during the two Battles of Fallujah, the first in April of 2004 and the second in November of that same year. In the first battle they just did it plain wrong and marines were killed.

In the months following the fall of Saddam Hussein in early 2003, Fallujah was one of the most peaceful and pro-American cities in Iraq. In April of that year, a crowd defied a local curfew and the protest escalated, with gunmen reportedly firing on U.S. troops. Soldiers of the 82nd Airborne returned fire, killing seventeen and wounding over seventy. When there was a review of the allegations of firing on U.S. troops it was discovered that no U.S. soldiers had been killed or wounded. But after all the civilian killings the attitude towards the American troops changed dramatically. In February of 2004, control of Fallujah was turned over to the First Marine Division. In retrospect it was probably a bad decision.

In March, four U.S. contractors were ambushed on the streets of Fallujah, pulled from their cars and killed, their bodies mutilated and burned, and what remained of the burned bodies hung from the city's street lamps. The Bush Administration, furious about the attack on contractors, unleashed the Marines. It did not go well. Tom's unit was not in that fight, but the Marines did what they always do, and as they fought their way into the center of the city they killed a lot of insurgents, but also apparently killed a large number of civilians even as they took significant casualties themselves.

It was brutal street-to-street, building-to-building, and room-to-room fighting. Marines were shot at from windows and alleyways. They were shot at as they kicked in doors and hurried across intersections. The AK-47s had poor sights and so weren't very accurate, but the RPGs at close quarters were deadly. No one, marines or insurgents, gave anyone a break. A lot of marines were shot at close range and the choppers couldn't get into the narrow streets to get them out.

These were the old-fashioned penetrating head and chest wounds. You were dead as soon as you were hit. The armored vests didn't prove as effective as advertised, the Kevlar plates had gaps between them so that, if you were hit by the shrapnel from an RPG or by enough rounds, you could get pretty messed up while the blasts themselves could leave whole squads dizzy and confused. You couldn't hear very well after one of those went off, and you couldn't think all that well either. And the insurgents didn't run away. They stayed and fought until they were killed. It was a mess, with the marines giving as good as they got, but it had definitely been tough going. According to some of the medics that Tom talked to about the battle, the numbers of deaths were a surprise.

The ferocity of the battle did indeed surprise everyone, but apparently no one more than those in Washington. It was as if they hadn't expected the damage or the casualties. The Iraqi Government, as shocked as Washington by the ongoing violence and increasing collateral damage, formally requested that control of the city be taken away from the Marines and turned over to an Iraqi local security force. There were those in the military who were convinced that the damage done to the city and the casualties didn't fit in with the Bush Administration's pronouncements that the war was over and the mission accomplished, so the offensive was stopped and the Marines pulled back and the city put under control of the Iraqi security forces.

Within weeks, those insurgents who had slipped away were back in the city, reestablishing their control and a presence that continued to grow over the next few months. The dangers from this resurgent center of the rebellion became too great and too obvious to ignore, and by September of that year, the city, as well as the whole surrounding Al-Anbar Province, was again slipping away from both the Iraqis and the Americans.

By October it was obvious that the Marines had to go back. The insurgents had weeks to prepare for the battle. Large numbers of booby traps and IEDs had been constructed and set in place, and throughout the city elevated sniper positions were created along heavily fortified defenses along the major entrance and exit routes. The Air Force and satellite photographs indicated that the return action would not be easy. But even facing the insurgents resistance during this second battle of Fallujah, the Marines did it right, with two different RCTs leading the push into the city.

On November 7, 2004, three days after the American Presidential election, a diversionary attack on the western side of the city was made to draw off insurgents from other parts of the city. The main attack came through the southern part of Fallujah. The two Marine Regimental Combat Teams, as well as a number of heavy battalion-sized Army units, along with British troops, were part of that offensive. There was intense bombing before the attack, and this time they brought up their tanks while self-propelled 155-mm howitzers fired at dug-in insurgent positions throughout the city.

After nine days of bitter and relentless fighting, the Marine Command described actions as mere mopping up, even though sporadic fighting continued until the end of December. A total of ninety-five marines were killed and over five hundred wounded.

But during the three weeks of the second Battle of Fallujah, the majority of insurgents were killed and as collateral damage, the city basically destroyed. During those weeks, the Marines were engaged in the heaviest and bloodiest urban combat since the retaking of the Vietnamese Northern city of Hue following the Tet Offensive. You could, following the Marines retaking of Hue, stand on the eastern shore of the Perfume River and looking out over the battered city, not see a wall left standing that was over three feet high. It was much the same in the retaking of Fallujah. Most of the city was turned to rubble but over 4,000 insurgents were killed.

The deaths and the wounds were different from that first battle of Fallujah. The insurgents were ready. Most of the casualties were from IEDs, powerful booby-traps, and even more powerful roadside bombs. There were numbers of burns that hadn't been seen before as Humvees and Armored Personnel Carriers were destroyed or set on fire. And there were also an enormous number of extremity wounds and traumatic brain injuries, as well as the concussive effects from the blasts, with five or six marines killed at a time and the rest of the patrol being blown apart, or coming out of those blasts deaf or blind and disorganized and confused.

During the second Battle of Fallujah, dozens of casualties who had to be massively transfused survived because of the use of whole blood rather than plasma, reconstituted blood, or blood stored for over three weeks. Virtually all who had been massively transfused did survive to be evacuated. The military's own data going back to Mogadishu, along with the experience of those who had to be transfused at the main military hospital in Baghdad early in the war, showed a survival rate that was over nine times as high for those casualties who received fresh whole blood compared with those casualties receiving the equivalent amount of blood divided into components or who received only red cells along with plasma or IV fluids.

But this time the Marines stayed. The city was destroyed but it was theirs. Of the 50,000 buildings in the city over 10,000 were little more than rubble. Every home had been damaged and over three quarters of the inhabitants had been displaced, or simply forced to leave. It was victory, but a victory similar to what the historian Tacitus said of the Roman Army. "They make a desert and call it peace."

Peace or not, the Iraqi Government could not hold the victory. By the end of 2005, the insurgents were back in control, not only of Fallujah but the whole of the surrounding province. None of it had made any difference. But after Fallujah, the tactics of the insurgents, whether Al Qaeda, Sunni, or Shiite, changed. It was a lot easier and a lot less dangerous to kill and blow up Americans from a distance without running the risk of gunships, fighter-bombers, and artillery.

Tom had noticed the change in their own sweeps through insurgent towns and villages. Before Fallujah, his tank moved down streets with a squad of marines going house to house to check for weapons and insurgents. One time, a squad of marines entered a house and came under fire. The insurgents were hiding in the basement, shooting up through the floorboards. Most of the squad was killed or wounded within minutes of entering the house.

The rules of engagement had been quite clear: any tank rounds were to be used sparingly with every effort to limit collateral damage, but they were to be used. As soon as what was left of the squad exited the house carrying the dead and wounded, Tom's tank put three rounds into the building, sending rocks, debris and shrapnel careening down the street and through the neighborhood. The rounds killed everyone inside the building. After a few minutes, the tanks and the grunts moved on. Leveling the building probably saved the marines coming up behind them, but it didn't win them any friends on that street.

But after Fallujah, the insurgents started placing the IEDS in the center of the road with pressure plates as detonators along the curbs. And the IEDs were bigger and more powerful. The roadside bombs had been just that, roadside bombs, when they were detonated they might blow a track off a tank or destroy one of the wheel mounts, but little else.

Now these bombs were exploding under the vehicles. And they were clearly setting the pressure plates to by-pass the lighter vehicles and catch the heavier APCs and tanks. It was a real surprise to everyone. The first time it happened, the force of the blast was so great that it warped the six-inch steel plates along the bottom of one of the tanks. People being thrown around and the blast wave itself had wounded everyone inside. The insurgents had clearly learned something in Fallujah. Nowhere was safe anymore.

As for dying, Fallujah had changed that too. It had been a long time since Vietnam. But there it was again: that crazy aunt in the attic, hidden away and barely discussed or even acknowledged but still able to make her presence known. The older sergeants, and certainly the field and general grade officers, would occasionally have mentioned Vietnam during training and even during Tom's first few weeks in Iraq, but after Fallujah, it was a lot more often, if not in a slightly more hushed voice.

Sudden unexpected kinds of dying were an almost daily occurrence now. There's not that much an eighteen-year-old thinks, or can even say, about death. Few in an RCT ever think of deaths, their own deaths anyway. They might think about being wounded, but not being killed. When you are young and in the Marines, dying is for someone else. That is a virtue, but it is also a mistake.

But with more and more IEDs going off in more and more towns along more and more highways and roads, friends and comrades who had been there in the morning were gone that night. That seemed wrong. Tom missed them all and was troubled that somehow he knew something important, even crucial, that none of their families knew, that no one who had cared for or loved them or waited for them, knew. It was all out of balance that he should know something so important that their families didn't know. But with a war to fight, the real meaning of those deaths would come to him later.

There was a grimness that settled in with the increasing casualties. Some of the grunts in the unit became angry. But the sweeps continued and more marines were killed and even more wounded, but they were also killing a lot of Iraqis. As far as Tom could see, probably as many good guys as bad guys.

At a routine roadblock one of the other platoons had set up late one evening, a car, turning a corner, didn't stop. It was dusk and difficult to see, but the car simply kept moving. A fairly large car bomb could kill or mess up anyone within fifty meters of the blast. There was never a lot of time at checkpoints, so when the car, ignoring the hand signals and whistles of the marines, seemed to speed up, the Humvee along with the tanks blocking the intersection opened fire. The 50-caliber machine guns tore the Toyota apart. Inside, they found a family, a mother and three young girls, killed, the fully jacketed high-velocity rounds having blown them apart. None of them knew what to do. So they left the car where it was and, clearing the checkpoint, simply kept going.

There were weeks now, as they moved on from dawn to dusk, where one town and village merged with the next until an IED would go off and they would level a house, street, or perhaps a whole block. They began to sleep next to their tanks and didn't shower for weeks at a time. There were days when supplies could not get through and they had to cut to half rations. There were even times when they worried about having enough gas for their tanks just to keep going. Fuel had to be trucked overland by tankers and, often those tanker convoys had been hit. There were barely enough troops to do the fighting, much less guard the increasingly longer supply lines. The insurgents could hit one or two tankers, set them on fire, and strand a whole column for hours.

There were rumors too, that the insurgents had begun hanging their IEDs from the overhead lampposts that lined the major town's main streets and boulevards. When they blew, the explosion and shrapnel rained down instead of up, killing or wounding everyone who had started to ride on top of the armored vehicles to be protected from the IEDs buried in the ground. Tom heard that they had actually blown the heads off drivers who were using the opened forward hatches of the armor to steer their tanks and APCs. If it was true, they certainly would be killing anyone manning the 50-caliber machine guns on the top of the Humvees or any of the other 50-caliber mounted vehicles. Tom didn't know if any of it was true, but it was enough that it might be.

Gradually the letters home, the email and even the satellite phone calls, became the same. Despite the increasing numbers of casualties, everyone, including Tom, always said things were fine, that they were OK and that, if not quite winning, they weren't losing either. But mostly the marines told their parents, their husbands, wives, and even their kids, not to worry.

But the whole country seemed up for grabs. There were armed guards and militias everywhere. You couldn't tell who was who, and certainly couldn't figure out who was on your side and who wasn't. Tom was sure that they killed a lot of people who shouldn't have been killed. He was sure they weren't making any friends. You could see it on the faces of the people in the different towns and villages they drove through.

What baffled him was the whole security contractor thing. They were everywhere. He could understand having private contractors driving the tankers; the Iraqis needed jobs; but having heavily-armed private security guards in the middle of a confusing war only made it even more confusing. One of the older grizzled master-sergeants told him, with the usual low-keyed mixture of both hostility and indifference so much a part of a lifetime Marine NCO, that there were somewhere around 60,000 independent security guards working for a number of U.S. companies that had contracts with the Pentagon or State Department in order to protect government employees and diplomats, or for just guarding things. "And a lot of the ones in charge are ex-NCOs with a couple of years experience and why not," he added drily, "an E-6 with eight to ten years experience gets around 50,000 dollars a year with hazardous duty pay working for the country, while that same sergeant working for one of these companies can get upwards of 150,000 dollars a year tax free. That's O.K. pay even if you have to work all day with a bunch of macho idiots and bottom feeders."

And that was the problem. These beefy mostly ex-military men with their beards and flack vests carrying government-issued M-4s and M-16s did what the Marines did without any obvious supervision and apparently no rules of engagement. They pretty much did what they wanted to do, including in some cases getting involved with the U.S. forces in their own firefights. Tom could see for himself that there were more contractors than military in some areas and that they had absolutely no accountability for what they did or didn't do. Apparently the military, not having enough troops, needed them, or someone thought they were needed. But it confused all the confusing things even more and certainly didn't lead to any sense of respect for the regular U.S. forces. It didn't matter if you were shot up or had a friend or family member killed by a contract security guard or a marine—an American was an American.

Tom actually heard that a squad of marines had joined in a chase—along with coalition forces and Iraqi police—of a convoy of these contract guards that had been shooting up cars and into homes along a major street in Mosel, finally stopping the convoy by shooting at the black SUVs that had become the signature of these security companies. It seemed to Tom that these amateurish trigger-happy private security contractors were screwing things up for everyone, including the Marines. It was crazy and everyone knew it, but nobody seemed to be able to stop any of it.

Not sure exactly what his own parents were hearing at home, Tom tried to write or send an email home every day. For the most part, he would write about the other marines in the unit, how they were all doing what they'd been trained to do, how they made sure they took care of each other as well as taking care of themselves. That seemed enough. You don't lie in the Marines. But you don't have to tell the whole truth.

They pushed their tanks well past maintenance guidelines. They had no choice. There were no tanks left in reserve, they were forced to just keep moving with what they had. But the constant wear, as well as the sand and dirt that got into everything, began to cause breakdowns. The heat only made it all worse. By midday you could fry an egg on the tank's armor plate. After nine weeks, the hubs on the drive wheels and the main bolts holding the wheels to the treads would begin to lock up.

Late one morning, they had to pull over and work on the gear train. Exhausted, having pushed on for days, Tom and the gunner, grim and drained, took the main spanner out of the toolbox. Climbing down from the tank, they started to work on the hubs. A couple of grunts set up a mini-roadblock at the nearest intersection to give them some cover. Pressing down on the back of the spanner for leverage, the head of the spanner slipped off the hub, shearing a piece of metal from the neck of the bolt. There was a moment when the pain left Tom stunned. A spasm of nausea swept over him as he grabbed his face and fell to the ground.

Even weeks later, it would be impossible to know exactly what happened. It could have been anything—a heat-expanded bolt, an overworked bearing, not wearing the prescribed eye protection, too much force on the spanner, a weakened piece of metal from weeks of taking the occasional sniper round denting the rotor mounts. But a piece of metal had come loose and tore through his left eye.

A Humvee took him to an FST, a Forward Surgical Team, set up about a kilometer outside the town they had just swept. The surgeon examined his eye and, putting on a simple bandage, called in a chopper that took him to the 24th Surgical Hospital at Ballad, forty miles north-northwest of Baghdad. An hour later, his eye was patched and he was being flown to Landstuhl Regional Medical Center in Germany.

At Landstuhl, they sewed up the major laceration of his eye and within half a dozen hours he was on a C-5A with a number of other med-evacs to Bethesda Naval Hospital in Bethesda, Maryland. A CAT scan in Germany had shown metal fragments embedded in the globe of his eye close to the retina, as well as in the tissues at the very back of the socket near the optic nerve.

It hadn't been lost on Tom, listening to the doctors talking among themselves, that if it had been a splinter from a round ricocheting off the side of the tank or a piece of shrapnel from a mortar or a roadside bomb, the metal fragments would surely have penetrated his skull and entered the frontal lobes of his brain.

There was some initial hope that the retina had remained basically intact and that the globe of the eye that had filled with blood would eventually clear, so that some sight might return to the damaged eye. Still, there were problems outside of the traumatic injury itself. One of the problems was infection, another was getting out the fragments without making things worse.

The surgeons decided to wait, to give the damaged parts of the eye a chance to calm down while allowing more time for the blood to clear, to give them a better view and if necessary better access to the fragments. Tom was told the risks and the benefits of waiting. He did not call his parents. Once committed to the battlefield, the old world, if not gone, is clearly no longer of use. Familiar customs lose importance and familiar rituals their power. At age eighteen or thirty-five, a marine decides for him or herself.

Tom took a deep breath and decided to wait. When he finally did call home, it was only to tell his parents that he had been wounded, but that he was fine and healing and that the doctors were confident that he would be all right. But the doctors weren't quite right.

The vision in his eye did not return to normal. He could see well enough to get by. There was always a haze when he looked to his left and it was difficult to see at night or in the dark and distances were out if he closed his good eye. Besides, Tom liked what he was doing and while the Marines would discharge anyone who could not see well enough to qualify with a rifle, the Army was different and would accept for active duty a wounded Vet if that soldier could pass the physical and waved all disability claims.

Special Forces was even less concerned about disabilities. If you could do what they asked and passed all the physical and mental tests, you'd be in. They clearly understood that anyone trying to get into Special Forces had to have overcome something along the way and a little dimness in an eye was not viewed as a problem anymore than not being able to carry a 100-pound bag of cement up and down a hill with a 30 percent grade a dozen times before breakfast.

Three months after being wounded in Iraq, he was discharged from the Marines and a month later the Army accepted his re-enlistment and, pushed forward by his time in the Marines, he was able to apply and begin Special Forces training.

Tom quickly found out that he couldn't sight his weapons well with his bad eye, but no one seemed to care. There was still Iraq out there. The general view in the military was that the lid would eventually come off no matter what America did or how many troops we had on the ground. But that didn't mean that we wouldn't keep troops there for the next few years. And there was Afghanistan looming again in the distance. The Special Forces understood that they would need more well-trained and committed men, even those who might not be able to see clearly.

10.

SHELL SHOCK / THE SHATTERING OF MINDS

Armies are fragile institutions, and for all their might, easily broken.

—Joe Galloway, War Correspondent

Psychiatry and psychology have never had an easy time of it in the military. It is hard to convince an army that you are injured when there are no visible wounds. But there is a toll to wars that has not gone unnoticed. During the early years of World War II, one of every four soldiers evacuated from a combat area was med-evac'd out as a neuropsychiatric patient. Approximately half of the medical discharges granted during those years were for psychiatric disability. Whatever else might be said about the battlefield, it is a fearful place, not only for the brain but also the mind.

No army is willing to admit that war is a frightening, and at times, terrifying business. Going into battle or being in a fire-fight the first time is difficult enough. Doing that same thing over and over again can become an impossible task. During the Marines' brutal December winter retreat from the Chosin Reservoir in Korea, an exhausted and freezing marine huddled in a fox hole was asked by a correspondent what he would like for

Christmas, which was the next day. The marine answered simply, "Tomorrow."

The military understands that kind of dread and foreboding. The best of the field grade and general officers, remembering their own times on the front lines, continue to feel it themselves. It was clear to those who knew of General Norman Schwarzkopf's history as a twenty-four-year-old captain in Vietnam and adviser to a South Vietnamese Ranger Battalion, that his refusal, during the 1991 Persian Gulf War, to let the Marines land on the heavily-mined beaches of Kuwait, was because of his own paralyzing experience in the Central Highlands of Vietnam.

In the spring of 1965, he and a company of South Vietnamese Rangers walked into a VC minefield during a night attack. The first they knew they were in a minefield was when Rangers started blowing up across the skirmish line.

Those who survived the initial blasts, including the future General of the Army, had to work their way inch by inch, slowly and painstakingly, on their bellies, feeling in the darkness with knives and bayonets for a wire or detonator, friends and comrades dying around them. It took those who survived, including Schwarzkopf, all of the night and part of the next morning to clear the field.

When asked by a reporter at a press briefing following the first days of Desert Storm why he had not let the Marines come ashore, Schwarzkopf snapped angrily, "Have you ever been caught in the middle of a mine field and had to work your way out of it?" Schwarzkopf, as Commander and Chief, was simply not going to let his Marines go through what he had gone through some forty years earlier. Instead, the Marines were used solely as a decoy. General Schwarzkopf remembered. Everyone in combat remembers. The only question is how personally they remember and how deeply.

Yet, no army wants to lose its soldiers because of something as universal and as apparently vague and personal as fear. It is not a soldiers' fear that worries the military. Everyone who has been in combat understands that much about war. What worries the military is that the individual fear might spread and become a kind of contagion that will lead to large numbers of troops simply giving up or refusing to go forward.

In the same way that physical wounds are easily seen and easily explained, military leaders have always tried to dismiss the anxiety and desperation of the battlefield as something physical. They have explained away those fears as something that *happens* to soldiers; something that is palpably real and not something that is either fanciful or what soldiers do to themselves. It is explained away as something physical, it is treatable, not something that can mysteriously spread to other soldiers.

The Greeks took a more reasoned, as well as a more humane view. In the Fifth Century B.C, the Greek historian Herodotus tells of a Spartan Commander who excused soldiers, though of proven bravery, who were "out of heart and unwilling to encounter danger." Herodotus also mentions a soldier called "The Trembler" who hung himself after a major battle.

At the beginning of the Civil War, the first war after the industrial revolution, where there was universal slaughter on an industrial scale, thousands of Union soldiers were suddenly diagnosed as suffering from nostalgia. It was a term coined during the Seventeenth Century to describe psychiatric disorders being experienced by civilians when they were far from home, but was quickly generalized to mercenaries, and then regular armed forces fighting distant wars. The idea was generally held by physicians during our Civil War that a soldier from Pennsylvania marching through Texas or Georgia could become so homesick that he would suddenly become dysfunctional.

But as our Civil War continued, the ferocity of the fighting grew worse and the carnage ever greater, with tens of thousands dying or being wounded within hours of the beginning of a major battle. An increasing number of soldiers, unwilling or unable to continue to go forward or becoming lost in the middle of the chaos and bloodshed, stirred the military and its physicians to find something more dramatic to blame as an answer for the trembling and fear than simply being homesick.

Those soldiers were finally given a definitive physical diagnosis. They were suffering from an "Irritable Heart." No need for magic here; no need to conjure up missing familiar places, malingering, satanic possessions, or cowardice. No need for any sense of personal failure or public embarrassment. The problem, whatever the symptoms, was clearly physical, the end result of an overly-stimulated heart. When the hearts of these men were examined, the hearts were indeed racing.

The shift in "diagnosis" did not make sense. Even to the most casual observer, the bizarre behaviors, including the psychological symptoms of depression, agitation, inability to sleep, mental confusion, and terrible startle reactions, appeared to have little to do with the actions of an ailing heart.

In World War I, that diagnosis was changed. The explosions themselves were said to create "shell shock." By 1915, those soldiers, shaken and trembling, removed from the brutality of the trenches, but still filled with dread, unable to sleep as well as to function when awake, were given the diagnosis of "shell shock." The medical focus had finally shifted from the heart to the brain and central nervous system.

By the beginning of the Twentieth Century, damage to the brain made more sense. The brain had clearly been damaged, shocked by the close proximity to the ongoing and unrelenting barrages of exploding shells that had become so much a part of this new kind of static trench warfare. Those blasts were enormous and they were continuous.

If a soldier came out of a battle or bombardment unwounded, but disoriented, paralyzed with fear, or simply unable to go on, he was diagnosed as having been too close to the shelling. The symptoms were the result of neurological damage caused by exposure of the body to the created shock waves. The blasts themselves didn't have to be explained. After all, anyone under a bombardment could feel the force of the exploding shells.

There were documented deaths in the Civil War and during World War I from artillery bombardments where the soldiers were found dead without any obvious wounds. If large explosions could actually kill a soldier without leaving a mark on his body, then certainly smaller blasts could injure the body's most delicate organ, the brain. The diagnosis was obvious. The soldiers' brains had clearly been seriously rattled.

It was, of course, a handy theory. If the shell-shocked patient recovered, the concussion had not been very severe. If the soldier did not fully recover, the damage was considered to be more extensive, but not severe enough to be permanent; if the patient never improved, the initial injury had been severe enough to be irreversible. If the patient intermittently lapsed back into bizarre or depressive behaviors, the damage was said to lie somewhere between the two different extremes. Once again, the importance of a physical diagnosis was that the soldier himself was not at fault, while the army, the family, and the country were spared the onerous task of accusing one of their own of cowardice.

Yet, during the "Great War," even that diagnosis did not stop some three hundred British soldiers, many clearly suffering from "shell shock," from being executed for cowardice. Though in 2006, the United Kingdom did finally grant those soldiers, and of course their families, posthumous pardons.

Still, it was difficult to admit to the crippling psychological effects of the battlefield during the Civil War, World War I, World War II, Korea, or Vietnam, as it is now.

Like all parts of medicine, from infectious diseases to neurosurgery, psychiatry too—along with its theories of mental illness—developed and progressed throughout the 1920s and 1930s.

Faced with the new understandings of psychology, less fashionable ideas about battlefield stress were proposed, though there remained the desire to maintain a completely physical version for those soldiers who simply could not continue. And for another sixty years, the physical explanations won out, even though symptoms continued to occur in soldiers not exposed to exploding shells nor those who had not been involved with sustained combat.

In World War II, the symptoms, along with the diagnosis of "shell shock," simply and quietly morphed into "battle fatigue." Fear and anxiety was now the result of physical exhaustion, of having been out in the field too long. A little rest, a little R & R and all would be well again.

In 1943, U.S. Army Lt. General George Patton visiting wounded soldiers in a hospital in Sicily, asked a wounded soldier to describe his injuries. When the soldier explained that it was "his nerves," the General slapped him across the face and called him a coward. It is a view that continues today, among those officers and enlisted personnel, who despite severe symptoms of PTSD, refuse to seek medical or psychological help for fear it will detrimentally affect their military careers.

Still, the idea of battle fatigue was carried forward into Korea, with its hard hills and even harder winters, morphing within a year of the beginning of the conflict into "combat exhaustion."

Sleep deprivation was now presented as a large part of the whole picture. Once again, there was nothing ominous or mysterious going on. Once again, exhaustion was something that was understandable and acceptable to those afflicted, to the culture, and to society in general. The stress of war was nothing more than fatigue, exhaustion, sleep deprivation, and a difficult job. Everyone could relate to that.

With the successes of Freud and the psychoanalytical movement, the diagnosis of "combat neurosis" began to creep into the military vocabulary, having replaced "combat exhaustion" by the time of Vietnam. There were now concerns about personality disorders, deep-seated anxieties, and unresolved childhood conflicts.

The conviction grew that there was something more complicated going on here than mere fatigue or exhaustion. It was believed that the routine short-term evacuation of these "stressed" patients from the front lines was not part of the cure, but a large part of maintaining, as well as adding to, the symptoms.

Guilt at evacuation, of not doing one's duty, of leaving friends and colleagues to fight on alone, was believed to play a major role in fixing the physical, and what were finally realized to be the psychological, signs and symptoms of the disorder.

The psychoanalysts proposed that soldiers surviving, while others died, could and did turn a few minutes of doubt, panic, and finally guilt into lifelong disabilities. It was considered best to treat these soldiers as far forward on the battlefield as possible, to maintain unit identifications and that, above all else, treatment was always to include the unwavering expectation, no matter how apparently tragic or disabling the symptoms, that these soldiers would be returned to duty as soon as possible.

The emphasis was to be placed on the previous health of the patient and not on the symptoms, on the soldier's ability to ultimately cope, and when appropriate, to acknowledge that for everyone the battlefield was indeed a difficult and scary place. There was clearly a mind to be considered now, as well as the brain.

By the time troops began moving into Vietnam in large numbers, the use of tranquilizers had become available. The basic treatment for battlefield depression, hysteria, and anxiety became the use of large dosages of the newly available psycho-pharmacological agent, Thorazine.

It made some sense. Neurotic behaviors deserved the new psychological medications. The idea was to drug these troopers, in essence to tranquilize them, in order to force them to rest, to let them sleep off their problems, and then gradually allow them to wake up, take a deep breath and, supposedly healthy once again, go back to their units.

Everyone quickly learned the drill. No matter what the symptoms, the treatment was always large dosages of Thorazine, rest, and being sent back to the unit. Whatever else might be going on, these patients were still members of their units, with the expectation that sooner rather than later they would all be going back to combat duty.

For the most part, it worked. At least the Army thought so. The more resistant cases, where even after they woke up from their drug-induced sleep soldiers couldn't function normally or remained truly disoriented, were sent to the military hospitals in Japan, Okinawa, or the Philippines. If necessary, from there they went back to the States.

But those troopers removed from combat were a decidedly small percentage of the large number of soldiers diagnosed with the newest combination of "combat fatigue" along with the new diagnosis of "combat neurosis" and all were treated with both rest and huge dosages of drugs. It appeared to work.

During the Vietnam War, the majority of patients with psychiatric diagnoses did go back to duty. During the whole of the war, 100 percent of soldiers with an initial diagnosis of "combat exhaustion," 90 percent with a primary diagnosis of "combat neurosis," 98 percent of the alcoholic and drug problems, 56 percent of the supposed psychotics, and 85 percent of the supposed exhausted and diagnosed neurotics, went back to their units with a bland, final nonjudgmental impression or diagnosis on their record of "Acute Situation Reaction." There were no ominous-sounding medical or psychiatric terms to disturb these patients, their units, their families, or the country.

And of course out of all of this, the military got what they wanted. The vast majority of those soldiers and marines were not lost to the fight. But there were also no follow-ups for those troopers after they were returned to duty. No one knew if they were the ones who died in the next firefight or, distracted and confused, called in the wrong artillery coordinates and killed their buddies with friendly fire. No one knew if they were the ones who missed the trip wire stretched across the path and, ignoring or not seeing the flattened area along the trail, tripped the mine or bouncing-betty and killed themselves and the trooper in front or behind them.

No one ever checked to see if these were the soldiers whose weapons jammed or went on to gun down unarmed civilians. And no one knew how many of these soldiers and marines who did make it back to the States would end up over the next ten, twenty, and thirty years in the country's different VA PTSD clinics, if they were lucky enough even to seek treatment.

But pain is pain. Once the Genie of the Mind is out of the bottle, there is no easy way of putting it back. Agitation, depression, guilt, mistrust, anger, thoughts of suicide, and emotional anesthesia, along with personal and social dysfunctions, are complicated multi-dimensional affairs. They can be persistent and, by themselves, can be more devastating than the loss of a limb, and as permanent as being blind or having a transected spinal cord.

What had always troubled the physicians and psychologists dealing with the emotional trauma of war was that these same symptoms occurred in civilian life—abused spouses who continually remembered and relived previous beatings, rape victims, abused children, and those involved in traumatic events like airline crashes and train accidents. They all had similar symptoms. It wasn't just war and it certainly had nothing to do with exhaustion or neurotic tendencies. All of it finally came together under the new and definitive psychiatric diagnosis of Post Traumatic Stress Disorder. But even with the diagnosis, it would take another thirty years and three more wars to finally begin to sort it all out.

But it is not only the increasing numbers of deployed military personnel being diagnosed with PTSD who have to be treated, the number of suicides among active duty personnel is also increasing. There have been a number of months since the invasion of Iraq and the surge in Afghanistan where deaths from suicide have exceeded the numbers of deaths from actual combat. It is not that the military does not understand or that they are confused about the cause of these deaths. The Pentagon's own data indicates that these suicides are the result of disrupted love relationships; that simply being apart, or worse, having someone pull the plug through a "Dear John" letter, can cause a soldier or a marine, away from home for months and sometimes a year or more at a time, to quickly spiral out of control.

What is known is that the majority of these suicides are best correlated to the lengths and the numbers of deployments, having little if any contributing factors due to combat. Suicides can and should be considered to be PTSD on steroids. But there is also the issue of prescription drugs.

The military medical system, both within the Department of Defense and the VA, has struggled to meet the demands of our two wars, and yet to this day still reports shortages of therapists, psychologists, and psychiatrists. But medications are available, and in that treatment gap the military has turned in ever-increasing numbers and in evermore complicated combinations to prescription drugs.

Across all branches of the military, spending on psychiatric drugs has doubled since 2001. Literally tens of thousands of troops struggling with insomnia, anxiety, alcoholism, flashbacks, irritability, chronic pain, and survivor's guilt have received prescriptions for sleeping aids, narcotics, anti-depressants, tranquilizers, and mood-stabilizers. *The New York Times* recently documented that many of these medications used together can cause severe and deadly complications. An Army report published in 2009 admitted the problem by reporting that one third of all troops deployed have been on one prescription medication, and of the 162 documented suicides of all active duty personal in 2009 over a third involved the use of one of these prescription medications.

Five times as many troops claim to have abused prescribed medications than admit to using illegal drugs like cocaine and marijuana. The truth about the actual numbers of suicides due to prescribed drugs may never be known, since those who are autopsied and are found to have multiple drugs in their system are usually given a diagnosis of "accident" as the official "Manner of Death." Whatever else might be said about our current wars, we are, as a nation and as a military, simply wearing down those few we keep sending back again and again to make the fight that is supposedly for all of us.

11.

THE WARS WITHIN

Post Traumatic Stress Disorder was officially recognized as a definitive psychiatric diagnosis by the American Psychiatric Association in 1980, when it was included for the first time in the *Diagnostic and Statistical Manual of Mental Disorders.* An official mental health diagnosis was an important step in finding unified answers for a condition that seems to arise from multiple and disparate causes. All the nonsense was to end. It was like when germ theory finally came to the study of infectious diseases.

The Army's goal though, has always been to keep its troops up on the lines, and where necessary, at the tip of the spear, while medicine's goal has always been to cure disease and relieve suffering. That on the surface the two would seem incompatible is only reasonable, but it doesn't have to be.

Larry Dewey, the former Chief of Psychiatry at the Boise, Idaho Veterans Affairs Medical Center and Clinical Associate Professor at the University of Washington School of Medicine, in his book *War and Redemption: Treatment and Recovery in Combat-related Posttraumatic Stress Disorder,* explains that it is the power of group solidarity, the love of comrades forged in the life-and-death crucible of combat, the binding and saving *esprit de corps* that keep the weak, as well as the strong, integrated within combat units, while keeping the majority of troops fighting on effectively whatever the circumstances and the ferocity of the fighting. There is a reason that the marines on their way to Iwo Jima already thought of themselves as dead and yet none gave up or refused to go.

Dewey points out that a study on bomber pilots published in the medical literature in 1943 documented that 95 percent of the 150 men who had completed their twenty-five combat missions over Germany and were headed home were suffering from what at the time was called "operational fatigue," and today would have been called PTSD.

Dewey's own clinical experience documents the large numbers of combat troops in recent wars coming home to experience intrusive thoughts of wars, nightmares, flashbacks, and hyperalert states, with little if any tolerance for anything that reminds them of battle or their former enemies. The issues of PTSD arise not out on the battlefield, but rather when these men and women come home.

While there are relatively few female veterans in the VA's PTSD clinics, Dewey and other VA psychiatrists are convinced that those numbers will increase over the next few years. Dewey has made it clear that the women in the military are strong personalities and strong people. You would have to be, to survive basic training and be deployed in combat areas doing combat duty. You were strong or became strong. "They will try to work through the problems on their own and right now that's what they're doing. But that kind of thing never works. The symptoms of PTSD do not get better and they do not go away. They will finally understand that much and will need to go into therapy. That's just the way it is."

Here is what Dr. Dewey writes in the beginning section of *War and Redemption* called "Descent into Hell." It is what everyone experiences who has been in combat and what all of us see in many of those who have made the fight and managed to get home alive and supposedly intact.

In this section, we explore the deep pain and burden of killing. We explore the role of propaganda in starting the killing and the role love plays in helping combatants wage war to its end. I portray through my patients' stories what the personal war of the ordinary combatant is like and the burden of guilt, grief, and pain that is carried afterwards. I present the deeper misery of killing civilians and other friendly combatants. Finally, we look at the forces that cause men (and women) to break down in war and afterward— overwhelming grief, exhaustion, guilt, and fear, in that relative order. We finish by clarifying some of the misconceptions that have arisen over the role of fear in combat breakdown and in prolonging the combatant's suffering through the rest of their lives.

Having to kill can leave emotional, moral, and spiritual wounds, that for many become the most troubling and most problematical results of war. *The Wall Street Journal* in 2005 got some of all this right. It was in an article above the fold published in October of that year titled "I'm not the Same Person." The *Journal* described what was happening to so many by documenting what had happened to one. That no one has appeared to listen is understandable; that no one seems to care is almost unbelievable.

This summer, Nate Self's wife caught him staring at his old Army uniforms, hung neatly in his closet.

"What was all this for?" the twenty-eight-year-old former Army Ranger asked. His wife Julie tried to reassure him. "Nathan, you did great, great things in the Army," she recalls telling him.

In January 2003, the Army Ranger captain sat in the Capitol as the President's guest while Mr. Bush gave his State of Union address. To the White House, Mr. Self was a symbol of American strength, resolve, and success in the war on terror. Badly outgunned, the young officer led his men through a bloody fifteen-hour firefight against al Qaeda fighters atop a remote mountain in Afghanistan.

After the battle, the Army awarded him the Silver Star, heaped praise on him, and assumed he would move swiftly onto the next war. He did. In the spring of 2003, he deployed to Iraq. There, Mr. Self began to suffer from grisly nightmares, anxiety, and depression.

115

Last year the war hero came home. In November, he quietly—and inexplicably, to his Army friends—left the military. A few months later, he was diagnosed with severe post-traumatic stress disorder.

Today, Mr. Self presents a different sort of model for the Army. He's a striking example of the emotional toll the wars in Iraq and Afghanistan are taking on soldiers and the U.S. Government's incomplete efforts to respond. Just as the U.S. military underestimated many things in Iraq—the insurgency, the need for better body armor and stronger vehicles—it didn't anticipate the levels of emotional stress soldiers have faced.

The medical path to the military aspects of PTSD began in 1947 with a paper by Kardiner and Spiegel, "War Stress and Neurotic Illness," that described a persistent, chronic and disabling war-induced neurosis consisting of nightmares, irritability, and a tendency toward angry outbursts, along with a general impairment of overall cognitive functions.

Half a dozen years later, an article dealing with a follow-up study of some 200 psychiatric patients who became symptomatic during the Second World War was published in *The American Journal of Psychiatry*. It reported the prevalence as well as the persistence of what, at the time, was still called "Traumatic War Neurosis." Physicians involved in the study continued to observe significant symptoms in these war veterans up to ten years after the end of combat.

A fifteen-year follow-up of these same Second World War veterans, along with the addition of Korean War servicemen, continued to document severe and persistent problems including startle reactions, significant sleep disturbances, and the avoidance of activities even slightly reminiscent of combat.

The Korean War veterans showed the same initial psychological profile as the World War II servicemen, with an increase in both the number and severity of symptoms in combat controls compared with the noncombatant veterans.

All the symptoms are treatable with group or individual therapy.

As Dewey points out, death or illness of close family members can activate war-related symptoms, the loss being too close to the pain of having lost beloved comrades in battle. Most veterans hate to get angry and try to avoid anger because it is so closely linked to many of their combat experiences and can trigger those intrusive war memories and feelings. But there are also those thoughts that keep veterans cautious about their relationships, always some version of the question, "If I really told them what I had done what would they think of me?" or "What type of man could do that?" The answer is usually self-condemning. All of this becomes more intense and more acute the older the soldier, particularly those with families and children of their own, and with over 40 percent of those being deployed to Iraq and Afghanistan being National Guard troops, that incidence, along with the severity of PTSD, has skyrocketed. Dewey has seen, in his own clinics, the hopelessness and concern of these National Guard troops increase with each new deployment.

And there is the whole issue of grief and shame itself. Those not in combat are forever embarrassed that others have had to make the fight, while those who have fought, and are wounded, know that others have been killed. There is no way out. This terrible parsing of combat can become a vicious and never-ending cycle where nobody wins no matter what happens. There is no easy way on a battlefield, where a few seconds of terror can lead to a lifetime of confusion and heartache.

But this is not just an American problem. PTSD is not restricted to any war or to any specific nationality. Symptoms and percentages of PTSD among Israeli soldiers who fought in the 1982 Lebanon war proved similar to those of U.S. troops in Vietnam, Mogadishu, and now Afghanistan and Iraq. PTSD is now viewed as a long-term, and in many cases, particularly if undiagnosed, untreated, or under-treated, a persistent and crippling reaction to the stresses of battle at any time or any place by anyone who pulls a trigger or sees someone else killed or wounded.

It is true that pre-existing psychiatric and psychological conditions, such as depression, antisocial personality, and alcohol and substance abuse, can be associated with an increased diagnosis of PTSD. But a high incidence of war-zone as well as battlefield exposures dramatically increases the risk of developing the condition in soldiers and marines without any pre-existing psychological conditions or anti-social personalities.

A survey of American soldiers deployed to Somalia supports this clinical observation. When the original mission of the U.S. troops in Mogadishu shifted through mission creep from humanitarian peacekeeping to the more familiar battlefield assignment of subduing a Somali warlord, there was an increase in the incidence of PTSD among those U.S. troops, with the greatest incidence in those exposed to both the physical dangers and the psychological trauma of actual combat.

The importance of combat in the development of PTSD became clear in a 1995 study involving veterans of the First Persian Gulf War. Deaths and combat casualties were blissfully light, but the prevalence rate for PTSD was 10.1 percent among those who experienced actual combat, compared with 4.2 percent in a matched cohort of troopers who remained in support units. It is expected that, with the ever-increasing exposure to combat situations among all the troops currently being sent to Afghanistan, there will be substantial increases in rates of PTSD similar to those seen in Somalia—especially as the campaign shifts from an occupation to the expected increases in combat as the Marines and Army units go after the bad guys as part of the new counter-insurgency doctrine.

All military data up to the present time, every meta-analysis of studies on wartime stress, collectively points out the critical issue of time on the battlefield as well as in combat as a precondition for the development of PTSD. That fact is already becoming evident in the most recent evaluations. The exposure to combat is significantly higher among troops currently deployed to Afghanistan than similar units now doing garrison duty in Iraq. Even in the oldest and more reviewed studies, more than 90 percent of those diagnosed with Post Traumatic Stress Disorder reported having been shot at, attacked by enemy combatants, or involved in some kind of deadly firefight.

Charles W. Hoge, M.D., in his article, "Combat Duty in Iraq and Afghanistan, Mental Health Problems, and Barriers to Care," reported a prevalence of PTSD of 12.7 percent among U.S. troops after they had been in three to five firefights, and of 19.3 percent after more than five. The author admits these are conservative estimates that do not take into account those most severely wounded. The incidence of the disorder can only be expected to increase as the number of troops fighting in Afghanistan and the desperateness of the battles and severity of the fighting continues to escalate.

The numbers injured, the severity of the current injuries, as well as the survival of those troops who would have been killed has only added to the incidence of PTSD among soldiers and marines deployed. A recent review of the psychological damage to our troops in Iraq and Afghanistan published in the *Journal of Massachusetts General Hospital* summarizes the problem:

Though the battle deaths for the current wars have been sharply lower than during past conflicts, the conditions of warfare in which troops must be on constant alert for roadside bombs and suicide bombers put soldiers at high risk of stress-related trauma. Moreover, many of the estimated 1.9 million troops who have been deployed to Iraq and Afghanistan are called back on multiple tours of duty. And with better gear and (better) medical treatment, they are more than likely to survive grievous injuries, with only one out of sixteen wounded dying, compared with a third of the casualties who succumbed in Vietnam and about two out of five in World War II.

Matthew Friedman, the director of the Center for PTSD, recently added to the discussion of the reason for the higher incidence of PTSD in our current wars:

Because of fantastic logistical support, med-evac capabilities, and medical advances, people who would have died in past wars are surviving their wounds, but they are at very high risk for psychological difficulties.

Despite documented increasing rates of PTSD, the true incidence may still be underreported. A retrospective report on PTSD documents what most in the military and those in the VA medical system already know. Of those whose evaluations are undeniably positive for a mental disorder, only 23 to 40 percent complained of or sought help for mental health problems while still on active duty. And those soldiers reporting the most severe symptoms were the least likely to seek treatment, for fear it would harm careers, cause difficulty with peers, be an admission of weakness, and worse, of cowardice in the face of the enemy. Soldiers trained to be tough and self-reliant are loathe to admit they have a problem, much less run the risk of asking for help. Experts estimate that no more than half of the veterans who would clearly meet the clinical threshold for PTSD ever seek treatment.

There remains the widely-held notion on the part of both active-duty personnel as well as those on career officer tracks that anyone who seeks help or counseling—even when they or their colleagues clearly recognize the severity of their psychiatric problems—will be stigmatized and jeopardize their own military careers.

In the military culture, "succumbing" to PTSD continues to be seen as a failure, a weakness, as well as evidence of not having the right stuff. It is a view that the present leaders in the Pentagon appear reluctant to challenge even while PTSD remains the most frequently reported problem noted in anonymous surveys among those soldiers returning from active duty in both Iraq and Afghanistan.

There is little doubt that those with PTSD who remain undiagnosed and so untreated, upon their return to civilian life, will fail at reintegration. It has been clear for some time that veterans who are diagnosed with PTSD have more divorces, more marital problems, and more occupational instability, along with the associated social dysfunctions, including higher levels of homelessness, more criminal arrests, and more acts of violence than do veterans without a diagnosis of PTSD. Without diagnosis and effective treatments, the psychological stresses of war never really end. With PTSD you can run, but you can't hide.

There are real future consequences of ignoring or delaying treatment. As late as 1993, a study of World War II Dutch resistance fighters indicated a sub-acute form of PTSD that had gradually become chronic: a delayed form of the disorder with onset five to thirty-five years after the end of the conflict. Israeli psychiatrists observed reactivation of PTSD among veterans of the 1967 Yom Kippur War when exposed to the news broadcasts of the 1982 Lebanon war.

But there is something more going on here that has added to the increasing incidence of PTSD among our troops, and that is the increased ages of those that we have rather indifferently sent and continue to send to Iraq and now Afghanistan. I recently interviewed a Norwegian Special Forces officer from the NATO Command. He was on active duty so he couldn't say very much, but he did say that he was surprised by the age of the soldiers that we sent to Iraq and Afghanistan. In short, he said that many were too old to take on the much younger and more nimble Taliban. He was obviously talking about our National Guard, which has always made up over 40 percent of the forces that have been deployed to the Middle East and are continuing to be deployed to both Iraq and now Afghanistan.

Not only are these National Guard troops older than the typical active duty soldier or marine, few if any are making or considering the military as a career. And yet, for many, the extended, as well as the second and third, deployments have not only exposed these soldiers to continuing combat situations, but have added to the burdens of combat, the stresses of families to worry about, and careers left on hold. War is always more difficult for those who are older and have personal commitments and responsibilities that go beyond their unit, their comrades, and even their own sense of patriotism.

The nasty little secret about the constant deployments to Iraq and Afghanistan is that the highest percentages of soldiers whose responses meet the screening criteria for PTSD are among members of the National Guard and Reserve units, and that those screening results are decidedly higher with each additional deployment.

Dr. Dewey recently wrote, "When you talk to many of these guys and gals who are constantly being sent back, particularly the older ones, you get an ever-increasing sense of hopelessness and doom with each additional deployment."

The constant danger, along with the so-called collateral damage of these wars, the deaths of women and children killed in bombing, during the large sweeps through towns and villages and at road blocks, have all taken their own unique and unexpected psychological toll on the older U.S. troops, particularly those who are themselves parents. It is this group who most experience flashbacks and late episodes of PTSD, after being confronted with the mangled bodies of civilians caught either in the cross hairs of the insurgents or their own weapons. But that was to be expected. War is always more difficult when you understand what dying and death really mean. It is in reality the old story about all wars. "If you keep going back, sooner or later they will kill you." Only now they can add PTSD.

What Dewey offers in *War and Redemption* is just that— both war and redemption. But in the process of dealing with these patients, he also offers a possible connection between the brain and the mind. He acknowledges what the Greeks and certainly the Romans acknowledged. The work of war is in the end, the work of death. And that the necessary killing is made immeasurably easier by the dehumanization of the enemy, whether it is as infidels, the gooks of Vietnam, the skinnes of Mogadishu, the terrorists of the world, the Nazis, the Japs, or the Ragheads. Yet in a very real way, killing is so difficult that the country has to work very hard to keep up dehumanization in order to get our troops to go back, again and again and day after day, to kill the bad guys.

The problem is that as time goes on and our troops continue to live and work in the lands of our enemies, these adversaries morph from the bad guys into insurgents and even freedom fighters. Some even become respected enemies, and as if that doesn't become confusing enough, there is the whole issue of collateral damage, the carnage brought about by that "Fog of War" itself. No one signed up to kill women and children, and yet these grim deaths become a nightmarish burden and even deep spiritual wounds, that can fester as much as those contaminated physical wounds. It is those deaths as well as the deaths of comrades that become the content of dreams, nightmares, and intrusive thoughts that can and do haunt many of our own returning warriors.

One of the major factors in the persistence of PTSD was missed in Vietnam, but is clearly understood today as a key contributor to the differing symptoms of the disorder. Recent clinical studies indicate that close to 50 percent of those deployed and returning home are not getting adequate sleep. They awaken involuntarily in the midst of the most disturbing battle dreams and nightmares. If they return to sleep they are only awakened again by the same nightmares. In the daytime, images of the grisly scenes of war intrude into their thoughts, making it hard to concentrate and focus, along with that creeping exhaustion of persistent sleep deprivation. Months and years of these symptoms predispose our troops to not just a full spectrum of PTSD symptoms, but depression and then substance abuse, as they self-medicate to try to find some relief from what more than one soldier or marine calls, "these war-cursed thoughts."

The question with all of this is whether these problems are physical or mental. Military and VA psychiatrists like Dewey lean towards the mind rather than the brain, but even they are beginning to understand that the mental has something physical to it. We remember things, which means that somehow those remembered memories have become fixed within the neuro-networks of our brains. Something physical has to happen to keep these memories current. After all, they are not happening again. They are being remembered. The idea is that if you can get beyond the nightmares you can get to the more deep-seated mental issues. And that is happening.

The work of Murray Raskind, published in the *Journal of Biological Psychiatry,* deals with a study of the use of an old blood pressure medication Prazosin, off patent now and so incredibly cheap, that easily crosses the blood-brain barrier to accumulate in the brain, and that, in the study of PTSD patients, can quiet the nightmares of these patients even as it improves sleep patterns and reduces intrusive thoughts.

Dozens of articles in the psychiatric and medical literature throughout the 1990s and first decade of the Twenty-first Century pointed the way towards a medication to treat the symptoms of PTSD. In 1998 Thomas Neylan, Director of PTSD program at San Francisco VA Affairs, documented in the *American Journal of Psychiatry* that traumatic nightmares and sleep disturbances were the most treatment-resistant and distressing symptoms among Vietnam PTSD patients. These nighttime PTSD symptoms contributed to alcohol and drug abuse, as well as suicidal thoughts, while precipitating completed suicides. The use of medications were rarely, if ever, effective in treating these nighttime symptoms.

Research studies indicated that specific receptor sites within the brain are associated with the emergence of these nighttime symptoms, suggesting that the medical blockade of these nerve cell receptors could provide relief from these traumatic nightmares and sleep disturbances, along with most, if not all, of the other PTSD symptoms.

Dr. Raskin's original paper using Prazosin as a specific alpha-receptor antagonist was in a cross-over study of Vietnam combat veterans. The medication clearly reduced PTSD trauma nightmares and sleep disturbances, as well as the persistent symptoms of depression, while improving the overall global clinical status, and in some cases even leading, for the first time in decades, to more typically normal dreams.

Raskind's clinical research at the Puget Sound VA and the Army's medical facilities at Fort Lewis, Washington, has been picked up by some of those who, like Dr. Dewey, are dealing with returning soldiers and marines, and like Dewey, are finally beginning to use the drug and reporting positive responses in both restoring normal sleep to today's returning veterans, while acting as a powerful antidote to the exhausting and increasing dangerous cycle of nightmares and intrusive thoughts. It may be the economic fact that the drug is off patent that is keeping the drug companies from actively promoting or disseminating this new treatment. In short, the drug as a generic is basically free to patients, so why would a generic drug be promoted nationally by the pharmaceutical industry?

But there may be another reason for the overall lack of use. As startling as it may be, the reason for its lack of use, or to put it less diplomatically, the refusal to prescribe it to PTSD patients, as reported by Robert Rosenbeck in the *Archives of General Psychiatry* in 2009, is that most of the clinical work on Prazosin has been done at VAs on the West Coast. Indeed, that is where Dr. Dewey practices, and medical information very seldom moves across the country from West to East. The influential centers of medical education and research are at the prestigious universities and hospitals in the East and, because of this, medical information moves across America starting in the East and moving West. Still, the published works of Raskind, Rosenheck, and Dewey, as well as the growing databases developing within the PTSD clinics of Oregon and Washington State concerning the therapeutic effects of Prazosin, have come none to soon.

But it is not only the increasing numbers of deployed military personnel being diagnosed with PTSD who have to be treated, the numbers of suicides are also increasing. In September 2010, the Pentagon released information that there had been more deaths in deployed military personnel from suicides than from combat. There have been a number of months since the invasion of Iraq and the surge in Afghanistan where deaths from suicide exceed the numbers of deaths from actual combat. And it is not that the military does not understand or that they are confused about the cause of these deaths.

Across all branches of the military, spending on psychiatric drugs has doubled since 2001 to over 280 million dollars in 2010 alone. The list of medications is extensive and in fact shocking: Prozac, Paxil, Zoloft, Celexa, Effexor, Valium, Klonopin,

Wellbutrin, Atavin, Restoril, Xanax, Adderall, Ritalin, Haldol, Risperdal, Seroquel, Ambien, Lunesta, Elavil, and Trazodone. We not only have the most powerful military in the world, but clearly the best medicated.

Literally tens of thousands of troops struggling with insomnia, anxiety, alcoholism, flashbacks, irritability, chronic pain, and survivor's guilt have received prescriptions for sleeping aids, narcotics, anti-depressants, tranquilizers, and mood-stabilizers. It is well understood within the civilian medical community that many of these medications, if abused or used together, can cause severe and deadly complications.

12.

Multiple Deployments / Brains at Risk

In Vietnam they would tell you that if you keep going back, they will kill you. In Iraq and Afghanistan, they say that if you keep being deployed, you will be brain-damaged.

—Conversation, PTSD Clinic, 2010

Both of the above comments are accurate. Indeed, the statement "they will kill you" was what Colonel Hackworth, an officer in Korea during the worst of the fighting and a colonel in the 101st Airborne following the Tet Offensive in Vietnam said to Joe Galloway, at the time a young UPI reporter who insisted on being part of many of the major battles of the Vietnam War. It wasn't said to be dramatic or to even keep the reporter from going back. That would be Galloway's choice. But it was a knowledgeable combat officer's professional assessment of the fight going on in Southeast Asia; no more and no less. It was reality.

The newer comment about being brain-damaged is also as accurate as it is insightful, if still lacking some of the overall acceptance of the facts. Again, it is reality—a new reality to say the least, but reality nevertheless. The reasons for these two different outcomes is the difference of forty years, the change in weapons, in strategies and tactics, in military medicine, and the fact that the insurgents in Iraq and the Taliban in Afghanistan, unlike the

Viet Cong and North Vietnamese Army in South Vietnam, are not so much shooting our troops as blowing them up.

And all this is happening with a medical profession becoming increasingly aware of how the brain functions, while growing more and more worried about the cumulative concussive damage following what may at first appear to be no more than minor or trivial head injuries. The growing connection between a concussion caused by helmet-to-helmet collisions during high school, college, and professional football games and the young men and women being exposed daily to brain-rattling blast waves from IEDs, suicide bombers, and roadside bombs, is too obvious to ignore. One cannot pretend that the exposures to recurrent blasts are not dangerous and damaging to the brain.

A recent University of North Carolina study showed that the average college football player receives over 900 blows to the head in a single season. In the pros it is even higher. In Iraq and Afghanistan virtually every soldier and marine is exposed to blast waves during each deployment and there are numerous Marine and Army units who have been deployed multiple times.

There are now autopsy studies that show that NFL players with early dementia do have significant anatomical changes to their brains and one would expect that much of the bizarre, if not anti-social, behavior of professional football players may well be the result of brain changes secondary to the repeated traumatic injuries.

In February of 2011, the former Bear safety Dave Duerson died of a gunshot wound. His death at age fifty was ruled a suicide. Duerson was picked by the Chicago Bears in 1983 after four years of football at Notre Dame, playing eleven seasons in the NFL, including two Super Bowls and four Pro Bowls. Experiencing bankruptcy and depression and apparently overwhelmed by the anguish of feeling that he was not the same person he had been, without quite being able to figure out why—so much a part of having a traumatic brain injury—he shot himself in the chest and not in his head in order to save his brain for analysis. Before he killed himself, Duerson left a message for his family to donate his brain to the NFL-supported Center for the Study of Traumatic Encephalopathy, a collaborative venture between Boston University Medical School and the Sports Legacy Institute that is engaged in research into the causes, progression, and characteristics of what is now called the "concussive crisis" in contact sports. If there is a potential crisis in contact sports, there is surely a concussive crisis in Afghanistan.

It is this whole issue of the cumulative effects of so-called mild sports-related concussive injuries that led to a first for the media. On Saturday, December 11, 2010, *The New York Times* reported that a rookie corner back had been arrested on a charge of felony sexual assault. What was different about the Associated Press report was the last paragraph. "The assault was said to have occurred after the player sustained a concussion …" What the reporter felt compelled to add to the article is ignored by the Government and the Pentagon. What is clear is that the accused player did have multiple helmet-to-helmet collisions. There is every reason to expect similar strange, if not dangerous, behaviors in those troopers repeatedly exposed to IEDS.

The researchers in neurology and neurosurgery, as well as neurophysiology, have predicted that the Twenty-first Century will be the century of the brain. The advances in real-time brain imaging techniques, nerve cell physiology, neuro-anatomy, neuronal receptor site analysis, along with reliable cognitive function testing, is beginning to bring to the study of the brain the same understanding that heart scans, stress tests, echocardiograms, lipid profiles, EKGs, and coronary angiograms have brought to heart disease and heart attacks.

That knowledge has proved so accurate and so universal that the husband who is a smoker, overweight, doesn't exercise, has a high cholesterol level, and who wakes in the middle of the night with "heart burn" and says to his wife that it must have been the pizza he ate, is simply ignored as the wife reaches for the phone and calls 911.

But actual brain damage from head injuries remains a contentious issue. The problem is what it has always been in medicine, that in order to have a physical cause for a symptom you need to find a physical change or some other measurable abnormality, anatomical or biochemical, somewhere within that organ system that is supposedly not functioning normally. You need a real cause to go with the observed effect. And that is where we now stand with brain injuries. The real issue is whether we have diseases of the brain or simply diseases of the mind, or maybe, like mass and energy, that the two are inextricably intertwined.

Occasionally in medicine, the history of a single person can best and most dramatically represent the struggle to first understand and then begin to cure a disease or treat a physical abnormality. Pasteur's history is the science of first discovering the cause of rabies and then actually treating the disease. Jonas Salk's and Albert Sabin's biographies are the story of curing polio. And in a very real, if less dramatic way, the professional story of Marilyn Lash is the history of brain injuries and the struggle not only to get things right, but to do something to treat, or prevent, the injury.

In the mid 1970s, Marilyn was a social worker in a regional hospital's rehabilitation center. At the time, the Vietnam veterans were being treated in VA hospitals and outpatient clinics. Very few of those soldiers and marines with significant enough brain injuries to have ended up in a rehab center survived to make it back to the States. The majority of them were usually killed where they were hit. But at the time, the rehab facilities in the States were beginning to receive significant numbers of civilian survivors of brain injuries. With the advances in emergency room medicine and trauma care, civilians were surviving serious brain injuries.

The early 70s had seen the development of CT scans to help diagnose severe brain injuries, while intra-cranial pressure monitors, measuring pressures within the brain and the skull, had begun to be used in the nation's neurosurgery units. It is the rapid rise in intra-cranial pressure following head injuries, rather than the initial trauma, that leads to the real brain damage and ongoing neurological damage, by compressing the brain and cutting off the blood supply and oxygen, causing brain cells to die.

The ability to monitor pressure warned physicians that things were quickly worsening. This allowed them to begin medical treatments to lower the pressure or to surgically remove any expanding blood clots surrounding the brain before any additional and irreversible damage to the brain cells occurred.

But survival did not mean a cure. The higher salvage rates meant that more patients were surviving but with more serious brain injuries and ever greater long-term disabilities. At times medicine can be a zero sum game. Most of these survivors were truly in desperate shape and needed all types of rehabilitation from physical therapy to occupational therapy, to cognitive interventions along with seizure control, and the prescribing of the appropriate psychotropic medications. The need for social workers to organize the rehabilitation programs for brain-injured patients escalated as the numbers of patients who survived significant injuries continued to increase.

When this was happening, the cost of care was skyrocketing. Insurance companies were increasing reimbursements for all kinds of medical services under, what at the time, were the basically unlimited fee-for-service contracts.

It was before HMOs and Managed Health Care. Insurance companies were issuing medical and hospitalization coverage much the same way that they handled car and home insurance; they simply charged premiums and then paid what was asked. That didn't last long, but it lasted long enough. A number of private for-profit rehabilitation companies, including some national chains, taking advantage of the generous reimbursements, entered the market, and with these companies in play and the influx of cash, there was an explosion of brain research as well as treatment programs.

Marilyn and others within the brain injury rehabilitation field were able to expand their programs and services, along with hospital stays that allowed comprehensive care, resulting in considerable improvement in the patients, as well as a growing sense of relief among family members.

But with the arrival of HMOs and managed care, reimbursements for hospital stays for patients with brain injuries went from an average of several weeks, and sometimes months, to under two weeks. Rehabilitation services in all their forms were drastically cut, with the care of these patients simply out-sourced to their families.

Marilyn Lash, like so many in the field of medical rehab, was unable to do her job. Frustrated with the growing gaps in services, along with decreased funding of virtually everything to do with hands-on patient care, she shifted from clinical social work to program development, hoping to get federal grants to continue some funding for rehabilitation programs. It was slow going but she eventually became the director of The Research and Training Center on Childhood Trauma at Tuft's New England Medical Center. But there was also a personal commitment to the treatment of brain injuries.

With the death of her parents in the middle 70s, she, and an older brother, had become responsible for the care and support of a middle brother who had suffered multiple concussions while playing both high school and college football. He eventually had to drop out of graduate school and, over the years, became increasingly disabled and eventually unable to live independently.

Marilyn had not only seen the professional lack of interest in brain injuries become a major medical problem, but was now having to deal with that disinterest personally. She had seen as a program director, as well as a caregiver, that both organized medicine and the health care industry would not address, much less fund or support, the long-term treatment needs of those with chronic conditions, including brain-damaged patients. There was no understanding, much less an acceptance, of the long-term effects of what were considered to be no more than minor con-cussive injuries.

Frustrated and angry, she experienced the terrible struggles shared by so many caregivers as they try to pull together ser-vices and supports within their local communities for loved ones abandoned by their physicians and their health plans.

She eventually tired of the cycles of writing grant proposals and reports for federal and state agencies that were ignored, and decided to go directly to the patients and their families. In the early 1990s, with her husband, Bob Cluett, who overcame a trau-matic brain injury as a child, she launched a publishing company that provided user-friendly, practical information to individuals, family members, and caregivers struggling with the results of brain damage and brain injuries. If the medical community, the health care industry, and the federal and state governments would not take care of these patients, they and their families would have to learn how to do it for themselves.

What Marilyn understood, two decades ago, and even more so today, was that the institutions dealing with the brain-damaged patient had become dysfunctional, while the brain injury research field, as well as the diagnostic and treatment facilities, had become so decentralized that everyone and no one was in charge.

Patients with brain injuries were under the care of neurologists, neurosurgeons, brain trauma experts, emergency room doctors, psychiatrists, psychologists, physiatrists, physical therapists, occupational therapists, speech and language pathologists and researchers—all doing their own thing. There was little if any coordination across disciplines or among experts.

Initially, the problem for brain-injured patients and their families had been diagnosis, and while that was in many cases still an issue, the real problem had become who did you call, or could you call, at two in the morning when things were not going well or as expected? The caregivers would not only have to learn the facts about brain injury as they were known, but they would have to learn the trade of brain injury care.

Marilyn and her husband formed Lash & Associates Publishing/Training Inc., a publishing house devoted entirely to making it easier to understand, help, treat, and live with brain injuries in children, adults, and veterans. Lash and Associates quickly became a leading publisher on acquired brain injuries and published individual research papers, while putting together seminars featuring the various experts in the many fields of brain injury. The company also developed an editorial board made up of academics who were leaders in the various fields of neurological disorders and injuries.

Lash and Associates became a cutting edge resource for both practical and user-friendly information on brain injuries.

The new business venture allowed Marilyn to maintain her own expertise in the administrative areas involved with brain injuries along with the newest advances in diagnosis and treatments while remaining focused first and foremost on patient care.

With the beginning of the Iraq/Afghan Wars, soldiers and marines began experiencing different kinds of shock wave brain injuries. The insurgents in Iraq and the Taliban in Afghanistan had switched from organized ambushes and frontal attacks to IEDs and roadside bombs targeted against vehicles and foot patrols. These casualties quickly become the largest and newest group of brain-damaged patients. They also proved to be the most problematical for both diagnosis and treatment and were initially ignored by the medical establishment, the military, and certainly the country. The increasing numbers of these patients made the decades-long efforts of Marilyn and her husband more timely and more important. Yet, even today, these damaged brains, along with their concussive injuries, have not yet been acknowledged as the signature injury of our latest two wars, even as they increase every day.

Marilyn and her husband have made it a priority to address these newest forms of battlefield injuries by publishing and distributing books dealing with battlefield brain injuries including *Down Range to Iraq and Back*, a book that contains information and resource materials for returning troops and their loved ones. *Once a Warrior* followed, dealing with the tens of thousands of troops who have shown serious stress reactions upon their return home, and that was followed by *Explaining Brain Injury, Blast Injury and PTSD to Children and Teens*. It helps parents explain the physical, cognitive, behavioral, social, and communicative changes that can follow a brain injury from a blast wave as well as the development of PTSD as a symptom of a concussive injury.

The number of brain injuries occurring in both civilian life as well as the military is astonishing, especially when compared to the prevalence of other diseases and injuries within the population. There were 10,000 women diagnosed with breast cancer in 2010, 75,000 men with prostate cancer, and 150,000 hip and knee replacement surgeries in what is obviously an aging population, Yet across America, during that same year, well over 2.5 million people were seen in private clinics and hospital ERs and given a diagnosis of Traumatic Brain Injury (TBI). 500,000 of these patients were hospitalized with over 50,000 eventually dying from the initial trauma and over 80,000 of the survivors going on to develop long-term disabilities. Many of these survivors will go on to suffer severe depression as a result of the TBI. Add to this mix the fastest growing number of brain-injured patients in history—the combat blast victims fighting now in Iraq and Afghanistan—and you have a sense of the size and scope of the problem. It doesn't help that blast injuries are clearly different and more confusing and longer lasting with a wider variety of presentations and symptoms than the usual civilian injuries— mostly falls, car accidents, and collisions on football fields—that result in blows to the head.

The Pentagon for its part has played down the ferocity of the fighting in Iraq and Afghanistan, but its refusal to acknowledge the growing importance of blast injuries as battlefield wounds is no more obvious than its refusal to award Purple Hearts to those with medically-documented evidence of concussive injuries from exposures to the blasts of IEDs. Indeed, at one time early in the Iraq War, the Departments of Defense, with the approval of Donald Rumsfeld, then Secretary of Defense, issued a moratorium on the release of all information regarding possible brain-damaged casualties, as well as those diagnosed with PTSD, among deployed active duty personnel, to any private organization or medical group.

The embargo of information extended to all public and private organizations, with a further restriction that these private organizations could not supply materials, nor give out any information or brochures, to patients or family members within any VA medical facility or outpatient clinic. Like so many of the official pronouncements about our wars in Iraq and Afghanistan, the reason for this moratorium was unknown and basically unexplainable. That embargo, however, ended with the shift to transparency under Secretary of Defense Gates and just in time for the 2010 surge of troops into Afghanistan.

The Department of Defense has become a major consumer of Lash and Associates publications. But just as the whole issue of AIDs finally came out of the closet with Rock Hudson's acknowledgement that he had the disease, it was the traumatic brain injury to Bob Woodward of CBS News in 2005, resulting from an IED exploding under his Humvee, that raised awareness of blast wave injuries among the American public. The spotlighting of Woodward on the evening news made him both the victim as well as the poster-boy for this new type of battlefield wound. The military could no longer ignore the fact that its soldiers and marines are being blown up and that damage from blast waves is a real problem, both for the troops and for military medicine.

Recently the Pentagon released information that puts the number of troops with TBIs since 2000 at slightly over 180,000. Those in the field of brain injuries view that number as preposterously low. A recent Rand Corporation report, challenging the official data, raises that number to over 300,000 of all deployed personnel. But the real numbers of those injured by blast waves are likely much higher, the result of what is now being called mild traumatic brain injuries or mTBIs. These are patients who suffer episodes of lack of energy, listlessness, emotional liability, startle reactions, surprising lapses of memory, reduced decision-making functions, along with depression and loss of word skills—any or all, without ever losing consciousness or having any evidence of a focal injury or any changes on a CT Scan or MRI.

These so called "concussive effects" are notoriously difficult to confirm medically and most likely account for well over 85 percent of all brain injuries in civilian and active duty military populations. What is important is that these concussive effects can become more severe and more persistent with each additional head injury, or in the military with each exposure to a blast wave from another IED.

Still, the military is particularly reluctant to acknowledge a neurological condition that can elude the current imaging techniques as well as sophisticated brain scans. Yet, these are the very injuries that may unfold slowly over the course of weeks and months, becoming the kinds of symptoms that family members explain embarrassedly to their family physicians "I just don't know what's wrong, he's just not himself anymore."

There is even a growing sense within the military's own corps of mental health specialists that the more serious TBIs, those accompanied with unconsciousness, may actually protect against the eventual development of PTSD by leading to an amnesia that protects against recalled memories and frightening experiences that could easily trigger the early, as well as the late, symptoms of PTSD.

What was becoming clear in Iraq, and even clearer now in Afghanistan, is that the brain's exposure to blast waves may be the most frequent and the most lasting of wounds. No one really knows the best way to accurately diagnose these wounds, or the best way to treat or prevent them. In the wars that had once been full of bullets, exploding artillery shells, rocket-propelled grenades, machine guns, chest and abdominal wounds, transected spinal cords, shattered livers, and fractured spleens there is something new. It is what Marilyn Lash and her colleagues, seeing the obvious, and refusing to look away, are calling our "Invisible Wounds."

13.

THE BLEEDING WARS

In its view, the "bleeding wars" offer the best opportunity to defeat the United States. Enlarging the war in Afghanistan is exactly what Al Qaeda wants, just as it wants the conflict in Iraq to continue ...

— *The Search For Al Qaeda/Its Leadership, Ideology and Future,*
Brookings Institutional Press (2009)

There was clearly no thought on the part of those who launched the attack in Afghanistan in 2001 and on Iraq in April of 2003 of our being bled to death, or that the Army and Marines would be stretched to the breaking point, and our National Guard pushed to the very edge of the cliff.

Iraq was to be a war waged on the cheap. As for Afghanistan, well, we did succeed in destroying the Taliban once and forced Al Qaeda out of the country, somewhat evening up the score for 9/11. If necessary, we could always go back and fix whatever was left to fix. Some ten years later, we still have over 50,000 troops in Iraq, with sectarian violence once again increasing throughout the major cities even as we begin to send more troops back into Afghanistan. Over the last ten years, the Taliban have returned to the mountains and plains of Afghanistan and hold more than half of that country, while the leadership of Al Qaeda remains intact in the mountainous tribal areas that border an uncooperative

Pakistan. What is clear today is that "Mission Accomplished" was no more than a snappy slogan.

Military histories written in the midst of the conflicts are notoriously incomplete compared to the less emotional, better-researched, and more-documented later efforts. But you don't have to wait to understand what went so wrong in Iraq and Afghanistan. Beginning after World War II, the military implemented what are called "After Action Reports" or AARs. These are the immediate and for the most part on-site interviews with the combatants and commanding officers following a battle in order to evaluate in a strictly tactical sense, leaving aside egos and politics, the conduct of a battle in terms of both the immediate successes and obvious failures.

AARs may be long or short, depending on the length and importance of the battle, but they are always informative. They act as a post-mortem, hopefully to serve as a future template to fix what went wrong and improve on what was done right. They are basically the authentic, unadorned, unrevised, and unedited history of what actually did happen.

Recently, a number of monographs based on AARs involving both Iraq and Afghanistan have been published in the military and foreign policy press. The most direct, learned, and unblinking of these evaluations were published in the *Journal of Foreign Policy* in the Fall 2008, under the bland and rather innocuous title, "Learning From Contemporary Conflicts to Prepare for Future War."

It was written by Brigadier General H.R. McMaster, who in the fall of 2008, as the Regimental Commander of the 3rd Armored Cavalry, finally retook the Iraqi town of Tal Afar, near the Syrian border, from Al Qaeda after three years of occupation by the terrorists. Looked at realistically, the twenty-five page monograph is not only a review of AARs covering the previous eight years of our two current wars, but its tone, as well as McMaster's position, is very close to the comments of the British military historian, Sir Michael Howard.

In his book, *Abuse and Use of Military Power*, Howard wrote, "While everything changes with the first shot, the key to any chance of success is not to be so far off the mark that it becomes impossible to set things right." Based on the AARs of the battles in Iraq and Afghanistan from 2001, the monograph is a professional attempt to begin to "set things right." While McMaster does not predict ultimate success, he does at least offer the way to keep us from fooling ourselves.

Here is the opening paragraph:

Flushed with the ease of the military victory over Saddam's forces in the 1991 Gulf War and aware of the rapid advance of communications, information, and precision munitions technology, many argued that U.S. competitive advantages in these technologies had brought about a Revolution in Military Affairs. Many argued that if these technologies were pursued aggressively, military forces could "skip a generation" of conflict and achieve "full-spectrum dominance" over potential adversaries well into the future. It was assumed that, based on the military technological advantages the United States already enjoyed, there would be "no peer competitor" of U.S. military forces until at least 2020. In the near future, it was assumed that U.S. forces would achieve "dominant battle space knowledge." Military concepts based on this assumption promised rapid, low-cost victory in future war.

These were the assumptions in place when the Iraq War began in April of 2003. It was the basis of the whole "Shock and Awe" approach that was to defeat the Iraqi military within weeks. As it turned out, the surprises were also on our side. But as McMaster points out, the battles a year earlier in Afghanistan should have made the administration, the Pentagon, and the country, suspicious of these new assumptions.

McMaster goes on to say:

At Tora Bora, for example, surveillance of the difficult terrain could not compensate for a lack of ground forces to cover exfiltration routes. After a 16-day battle, many Al Qaeda forces, including Osama bin Laden, escaped across the Pakistan border.

And later, when U.S. intelligence detected a concentration of Taliban forces in the Shah-i-Kot valley, commanders deliberately planned an attack that would include two American Infantry battalions reinforced with Afghan and other Allied troops. Intelligence prepared for the operation spanned two weeks. U.S. forces focused every available surveillance and target acquisition capability, including satellite imagery, unmanned aerial vehicles, and communications and signal intelligence assets, on a 10X10 km box that defined the battleground. Enemy countermeasures to the sensors, however, were effective, and the fight was characterized by a high degree of uncertainty.

As the fight developed, it became apparent that more than half of the enemy positions and at least 350 Al Qaeda fighters had gone undetected. The enemy's reaction to the attack also was unexpected. American commanders had expected Al Qaeda forces to withdraw upon contact with the superior force rather than defend as they did from fortified positions. The unit had deployed with no artillery, assuming that surveillance combined with precision fires from the air would be adequate.

However, even the most precise bombs proved ineffective against small, elusive groups of enemy infantry. In fact, soldiers (without artillery support) had to rely on small mortars. A combination of small unit skills, soldier initiative, and determined leadership permitted American forces to shake off the effects of tactical surprise, defeat Al Qaeda attacks on the landing zones, and then mount an offensive.

During these early battles the advanced surveillance and information technologies failed to deliver the promised "dominant battlefield knowledge" as enemy forces employed traditional old-fashioned countermeasures to these high-tech capabilities, such as dispersion, concealment, deception, and intermingling with civilian populations.

The Third Infantry Division, in crossing the Euphrates River, ran into an undetected Iraqi armored brigade that counterattacked in a failed attempt to regain control of crossing sites along the river. There were a large and unexpected number of casualties.

What is clear from a review of AARs is that these were not the wars, much less the kinds of battles, that had been planned for nor expected. The 1st Cavalry Division was actually sent to Iraq without its armor. As bizarre as it now seems, the Division off-ramped in Iraq with no tanks. But with casualties mounting within the Division and its units bogged down fighting insurgents within Iraq's towns and cities, those same tanks had to be airlifted into Iraq from the States, one at a time, aboard C-5As.

It is a fundamental military doctrine that without tanks any firefight becomes basically light infantry against light infantry. In those battles, the forces in control of the terrain, whether in cities or towns or along mountain passes, have the advantage of making the fight where they want and on their terms. In reality, if you have to go around kicking in doors or patrolling along narrow mountain paths, those behind the doors or using the rocks for cover always have the tactical advantage. That makes going on street patrols and setting up temporary road blocks in the midst of enemy forces while having to decide within seconds who to shoot and who to let go, at the same time that you are worrying about being shot or blown up yourself, is not only frightening but exhausting work. Do that every day and it quickly becomes impossible. And that is exactly what has happened and continues to happen to the majority of our troops.

The AARs dealing with the initial run up from Nasiriyah to Baghdad at the very beginning of the Iraq War point out that even back then the initial lack of troops was the cause for the ever-increasing numbers of casualties.

Troop strength compelled [our] dispersed forces to move continuously along routes that they were unable to secure, which, one could argue with confidence, was the principal cause of the large number of casualties from roadside bombs.

This kind of war, with not enough troops on the ground—leading to small unit firefights, ambushes of supply columns, the use of IEDs along with suicide bombers—has not only led to a startling number of amputations and traumatic brain injuries, but to a new kind of PTSD where deployed personnel returning home have flashbacks and anxiety attacks simply driving a car down a highway, and nightmares about going to a movie or walking down a crowded street. We can't do this without more of a national commitment and we can't do this without a lot more troops or we shouldn't even try to do it at all.

As McMaster points out:

In war, we have to reject the notions that lightness, ease of deployment and quickness are virtues in and of themselves. Forces must also have staying power and survivability if they are to succeed.

What unit commanders need to know most about enemy forces, such as degree of competence and motivation, lay completely beyond the reaches of technology. And military units, whether a squad, platoon, company, battalion, or brigade, have to be able to survive as well as fight. Out on the battlefield, back-ups do count and redundancies do matter. And that cannot be done on the cheap.

What McMaster documents is that our reliance—to the exclusion of virtually everything else—on technology and sophisticated weapons systems to control the battlefield is a flaw in both our strategic as well as our tactical thinking. It is an approach to warfare and the battlefield that can best be described as "Gadgetry Replacing Strategy." It puts every soldier and marine at risk.

Sir Rupurt Smit, a general in the British Army who won praise from American generals as commander of the 1st Armored Division in the First Gulf War, has offered much the same assessment, though in the less dramatic and decidedly more understated British way.

"Frequently we can see that our opponents deliberately operate below the threshold of the utility of our weapons and organization as we would wish to use them ... We have equated technology with the use of force ... but force can be achieved by throwing rocks ...

When a terrorist can detonate a bomb with a mobile phone our battalions are useless."

Yet, the real message in *Learning from Contemporary Conflicts to Prepare for Future Wars* is in the final summation. The ending is more than a cautionary tale and more than the difference between winning and losing. It is the difference between coming home intact or in a box, or with your arms or legs blown off, having a traumatic brain injury or a diagnosis of PTSD.

Wars cannot be waged efficiently. In both Afghanistan and Iraq, the United States' planned troop reductions assumed a linear progression toward stability. As a result, units shifted areas of operation to compensate for troop shortages and unit deployments were accelerated, as it became clear that "off ramp" plans were unrealistic. Moreover, a short-term approach to long-term problems generates multiple short-term plans that confuse activity with progress.

But perhaps Gladstone, the Prime Minister of England during the reign of Queen Victoria, who presided over the failure of the British invasions of Afghanistan, explained it best when, at the end of his career, he was asked by a reporter what was the most difficult part of being Prime Minister. Gladstone did not hesitate, "Why reality, my dear boy—reality!"

14.

IEDs / Blasts that Kill and Maim

Every war has its own signature wounds. At Agincourt and Crecy in the Fifteenth Century, it was the puncture wounds inflicted on the French knights by flights of arrows from English longbows. The beginnings of gunpowder-propelled projectiles, the muskets of the Sixteenth Century, led to chest and abdominal wounds never before seen on a battlefield, while the cannon balls with their explosive charges led to multiple as well as massively contaminated wounds that inevitably proved fatal.

In our own Civil War, it was high-velocity bullets fired with astonishing accuracy from weapons with rifled barrels that caused the new types of deeply penetrating and tissue-shattering wounds. The bullets hit with such impact that they routinely broke bones, leading to the thousands of amputations that became the hallmark of the major battles of the war, from Harper's Ferry to Shiloh, Spotsylvania, Antietam, and Gettysburg.

The Civil War was the first major war following the Industrial Revolution and the slaughter was on an industrial scale. By the end of the war, well over a third of all the men in the State of Mississippi had become amputees. And the carnage has simply increased with each new decade and each new war.

During the First World War, it was machine gun fire that caused multiple head, torso, and abdominal injuries. The majority of those wounded bled to death from punctured lungs, shattered livers and spleens, blown-away abdominal aortas, torn iliac arteries, and fractured kidneys. There was a reason that 20,000 soldiers died on the first day of the Battle of the Somme.

In the Second World War, it was multiple shrapnel wounds from barrages of artillery, as well as burns from exploding tanks, trucks, and torpedoed ships leaking tons of flammable fuel oil easily ignited, that were the major causes of both deaths and disabilities. The real lifesavers during those years of fighting in the fields of Europe and the jungles of the Pacific was the availability, beginning in 1941,of the newly discovered sulfur antibiotics, along with the use of plasma and other blood substitutes, as well as better and more effective wound care.

In Vietnam it was vascular injuries caused by booby traps and close-up machine gun and small-arms fire, exploding satchel charges, and shrapnel from rocket-propelled grenades. Those who lived survived because of rapid med-evacs to a surgical or evac hospital, the increasing skills of the surgeons, and the development of grafting techniques to reconstruct damaged arteries and veins.

Today, in Iraq and increasingly in Afghanistan, it is polytrauma and traumatic brain injuries from the blasts and shock waves of car, roadside bombs, and suicide bombers that have become the major cause of casualties and death leading to what are these war's signature wounds—amputated and destroyed limbs and traumatic brain injuries.

The sad truth is that there is little "improvised" in an explosion that can turn over a 70-ton M1A1 tank, blow the windows out of every building within a four-block radius, or rattle the brains of any soldier or marine within a dozen meters of even the smallest blasts.

In Iraq and Afghanistan, it is the powerful blast waves even more then the heat and projectiles from the explosions that does the most damage to internal organs, rupturing bladders and stomachs, causing air to leak from the lungs leading to asphyxia and sudden death, as well as injuries to the brain itself. Of all the organs of the body, the brain is the most susceptible to damage from rapid and dramatic shifts in atmospheric pressures, in short, from the shock waves generated by detonated IEDs.

What nature gives, nature often takes away. Placing the brain within the protective shell of the skull, while having clear evolutionary advantages, can be a real problem if the brain is set into motion from the head being hit with a hammer, a fall in the bathroom, or the passing pressure wave front of an exploding IED. Even thirty or forty meters out from the center of a large explosive charge, brain tissues can be significantly, and in some cases permanently, damaged.

The Pentagon's own data on IEDs is scary at best and terrifying at worst. Wire together three 155-mm artillery shells, put them in the ground and cover them with a few pounds of Centex, then put some canisters of butane gas on top of the explosives and the temperature at the center of the explosion will reach between 6,000 and 7,000 degrees. The blast wave moves at 1,000 feet per second with a pressure gradient of 400 pounds per square inch, or over a 1,000 times atmospheric pressure.

The blast waves of high pressure spread out in all directions, followed closely by what is called a "secondary wind," the result of the huge volume of displaced air flooding back into the area of low pressure generated in the wake of the original blast front.

Even if you manage to survive the flying debris and projectiles set into motion by the explosive charge, the concussive effects of both wave fronts are by themselves substantial and dangerous. Military physicians have learned that significant blast injuries should be expected in any soldier exposed to an IED, whatever the distance from the explosion.

The new U.S. German-style helmets with flared earflaps may protect against projectiles, but are not designed to absorb the force of an explosion. In a blast, the weight of these helmets only adds to the injury.

"It's like a pan on your head, held by a shoestring webbing," an Army combat engineer explained. "When you take a hit, it rings your head like a bell."

A 2005 medical paper on casualties resulting from blast injuries cautioned that such injuries are "notorious for their delayed onset." In truth, very few are spared the blast effects of a car or roadside bomb. It is the newest legacy of these newest American wars and a legacy that keeps increasing each month.

This susceptibility of the brain to the physics of trauma has to do with the unique way the brain is put together and where it sits in the body. Resting on the neck, it is basically hung out there in the wind, suspended within a rim of protective fluid inside of the hard, unyielding surrounding shell of bones that make up the skull.

Encased within the skull, the brain has no place to go when it starts to move either forward or backward, starts to swell, or becomes compressed from an expanding blood clot.

If you have a motorcycle or car accident on a freeway, hit your head, and manage to make it to a major trauma center hospital alive, the ER docs and the neurosurgeons know exactly what to do and in what order to do it. They will not only be able to keep you alive, but with a little luck, be able to save your brain, and by extension, your mind. Keeping the two together and intact is no small thing. Ask anyone who has to take care of one of the 1.4 million traumatic brain injuries that occur in this country each year and he or she will tell you how inseparable and intertwined the two have always been, a connection made decidedly more obvious once the brain has been injured.

As soon as you enter the emergency room as a "head injury," have your blood pressure and breathing stabilized, the ER docs, depending on the degree and severity of the injury, put you into a drug-induced coma to slow down any ongoing damage to the injured brain cells and protect any of the remaining healthy cells from undergoing any secondary or collateral damage. They will, if there is overt difficulty in breathing or maintaining heart rates, add a calcium channel blocker to help stabilize the outer membranes of the injured cells, while maintaining normal intracellular metabolism. If your blood pressure becomes too high, the ER personnel will lower the pressures to protect against any re-bleeding into the brain and the causing of more tissue damage. If the pressures are too low, they will add medications to raise the pressures to maintain adequate blood flow to the brain and central nervous system, even if an injury is present. But that kind of protecting against any ongoing brain damage requires great skill and constant monitoring and can, at its best, become a very "iffy" thing.

If the brain itself does begin to swell, they will start IV solutions of concentrated saline in the hopes of drawing off the accumulating fluids to control the swelling. If that doesn't work, they'll add an IV diuretic to drain the body of it own waters in an effort to keep down intra-cranial pressure. If the hypertonic fluid and diuretics don't work, they will take you to the OR and have the neurosurgeons remove the sides of your skull to allow the brain to swell without compressing and damaging any of the still-normal tissues.

Since the brain resides in a closed rigid space, the overriding idea behind removing parts of the skull is to relieve any increasing intra-cranial pressure that could further damage the brain. When the swelling has finally begun to resolve and the brain is back to normal size, the surgeons will simply put back the part of the skull that had been removed and wait for the patient to recover. It works and has worked thousands of times each year in emergency rooms and major trauma centers around the country and around the world.

But a brain damage from the shock wave of an IED is a different kind of injury. That first became evident when the usual treatments for head injuries didn't work. There is something unexpected going on down at the cellular or sub-cellular level of the brain following an exposure to a pressure wave that is not the same as getting hit on the head during a car accident or from a fall in the bathroom. We have a new kind of war and should have expected new kinds of wounds and causalities. Brain injuries from IEDs are different from all the usual kinds of neurological war injuries such as damaged spinal cords, penetrating head wounds, or skulls simply blasted apart.

And this new kind of war, with new kinds of wounds, is here. Roadside bombs killed 268 Americans in Afghanistan in

2010, a 60 percent increase over the previous year, even as the Pentagon tries to employ new methods to counter these weapons. The numbers of wounded by these weapons has also soared and is on an even higher trajectory for 2011, with over 3,000 U.S. service members injured enough to be evacuated from the combat areas. The problem in detecting these bombs in Afghanistan is that these IEDs are remarkably less sophisticated then the IEDs used in Iraq, typically relying on fertilizer and diesel fuel, these explosive devices made by the militants in Afghanistan cannot be scanned by electronic devices to jam their frequencies because these bombs lack the circuitry that make them easy to detect and disarm or destroy.

A bewildered neurosurgeon at one of the Combat Surgical Hospitals in Iraq was heard to say in early 2004 that he'd rather take care of a patient with a penetrating head wound, "that way there is only the damage along the track of the bullet."

Congresswoman Gabrielle Giffords survival and recovery following being shot in the head at the Tucson supermarket is a graphic example of the neurosurgeon's preference. Following the bullet entering the left side of her skull, the major damage to the congresswoman's brain was only along the path of the bullet. The bullet itself did not cross the midline of the brain, where it surely would have damaged any number of vital structures, not only connecting the brain's right and left hemispheres, but those areas necessary to maintain adequate respiration and normal heart rate. Apparently the speech center on the left side of her brain was significantly damaged, and the immediate surgery cleared away the damaged and dying tissues, along with any bullet fragments and pieces of bone and at the same time removing the blood clots, allowing the repair of any damaged blood vessels and hopefully limiting any further damage from infections or additional bleeding, giving the congresswoman the chance not only of surviving, but the ability to overcome what was sure to be significant speech, emotional, and cognitive defects. A gunshot wound to the dominant hemisphere is never fully recoverable. But the fact that the bullet was a 22-caliber round rather than a larger bullet helped to limit the type, degree, and severity of damage.

Had the congresswoman been in Iraq or Afghanistan and instead of a 22-caliber bullet entering her brain, she'd been struck with a large shock wave an exploding roadside bomb or IED, she might well have survived, but the injury to other parts of her brain rather than just the damage along the track of the bullet would have made any chance of a major recovery close to zero.

With a blast injury, you may have to deal with damage to most of the brain. Blast injuries affect more widespread parts of the brain than the typical shell fragment injury or bullet wound. It is an understanding that is shared by everyone involved with caring for a patient following a closed-head injury from a roadside bomb.

The irony, as so often happens in any new war, is that ingenuity can always trump traditional tactics and weapons. IEDs employed by the insurgents in Iraq and the Taliban in Afghanistan have become the low-tech answer of an enemy that lacks the firepower to confront a modern army and so becomes, not only the weapon of necessity, but the weapon of choice.

Strategically, IEDs have let the insurgents in Iraq and the Taliban in Afghanistan take advantage of our tactical mistakes. There were not enough troops on the ground in either country to offer real security, forcing our units to be constantly shifted from one contested area to another. That movement opened up the poorly-guarded highways and undefended roads to both ambushes and the planting of increasingly sophisticated, and more lethal, IEDs.

And all of this without forcing the enemy to concentrate their forces and run the risks from artillery, helicopter gun-ships, and bombing runs of low-flying fighter planes. In these untraditional wars, or what the military call "asymmetrical conflicts," the enemy doesn't have to win, they just have to not give up.

It is clear though that neither Al Qaeda, the Shiites, the Sunnis, or the Taliban had any idea about the intrinsic subtleties of brain function or the effects of blast waves on the higher cognitive functions, or even basic neuronal activity, when they picked the suicide bomber, car and truck bombs, and roadside IEDs as their weapons of choice. For them, the unexpected brain damage is no more than a lucky battlefield by-product of their kind of war. But for us and our own, these weapons have become a terrible problem, not only as a sledge hammer able to disable tanks and kill a dozen of our troops at a time, but the cause of a new kind of collateral damage that we are only now beginning to understand and may some day be able to treat.

The fact that the usual treatments for traumatic brain injuries turned out not to work as expected in Iraq and Afghanistan, came as its own kind of shock to the military neurologists and neurosurgeons. There were all kinds of initial but foolish theories about the neurological damage following exposures to the blasts, that ran from the release of tiny air bubbles within the micro-circulation of the brain following exposure to a shock wave, to damaging individual brain cells through some kind of cellular injury due to the inhaling of neurotoxic substances from the acrid smoke of the explosive charges themselves.

The point is that nobody understands why the brains of soldiers and marines exposed to blast waves do not recover. A Rand Report published this year stated that over 300,000 of our combat troops had been exposed to one or more IEDs during their deployment and those numbers do not contain the results from our latest "surge" in Afghanistan.

Civilian neurologists have always worried about the long-term effects of concussive injuries. But they drew comfort for themselves and their patients if the head trauma did not result in immediate unconsciousness or confusion, or if the effects lasted less than a few minutes, and amnesia for the event didn't exceed twenty-four hours. They drew even more comfort if routine CT scans or MRIs did not show any evidence of a significant anatomical injury, including hemorrhages or small areas of tissue swelling.

If the injuries fit those criteria, the feeling was that there was little to worry about and few long-term concerns, even if there were a few days of headaches following some initial nausea. A general consensus developed within the medical community that a head trauma patient without any initial obvious signs of significant brain injury and negative imaging studies did not have a significant "concussive injury" whether as the result of an accident on the freeway, falling off a bicycle, helmet-to-helmet contact on the football field, or being near an IED.

The standards for diagnosing a mild Traumatic Brain Injury or mTBI had been set quite high, which was comforting to everyone except patients and their families. But being comforted in medicine isn't necessarily being correct. What is now becoming obvious is that exposure to the wave front of an exploding IED is different from hitting your head during a fall, being hit on the head with a hammer, or being thrown from a car during an accident.

There was concern about this whole medical DWT or "Don't Worry Thing" concerning the long term effects of mTBIs, or what some neurologists insisted on calling mild concussive injuries. After all, there was the medical, as well as the fictional, literature on the punch-drunk boxer. Traditional medical views aside, being hit in the head has always caused significant and unexpected neurological problems.

During the 2008 baseball season, the center fielder for the Minnesota Twins, racing backwards to catch a fly ball, lost his balance, fell backwards, and hit his head on the Astroturf. The ballplayer experienced some initial confusion, which cleared by the next inning. The CT scans and MRIs showed nothing abnormal. But the player had lost his fine-tuned coordination, or at least the necessary coordination, to hit a ninety-seven mile an hour fastball. He was never again the hitter he had been before his head hit the Astroturf, and he was forced to withdraw from baseball at the end of the following season. Even seemingly minor head injuries can have profound and lasting effects.

There have always been those few sports medicine physicians who point out the absence of any concussive injury in contact sports where the players do not wear helmets. According to those physicians, the brain is not put in danger from the risky behaviors of the helmeted sports where the players launch themselves full speed and head first at one another.

Only recently has the National Football League documented severe dementias in former players at unexpectedly early ages.

For the most part these are players who had multiple helmet-to-helmet episodes during their college and NFL careers. A few such contacts may have led to symptoms of disorientation, as well as headaches, for minutes if not hours, yet the majority of these helmet-to-helmet contacts were simply shaken off and the players put back into the game.

The League has recently been challenged by family members, as well as some physicians, that the increased incidence of dementia in these professional players, the majority in their late fifties and early sixties, is out of proportion to the incidence of dementia in other men their ages in the general population. It appears that what initially can be dismissed as trivial head trauma—no loss of consciousness, no seizures, no persistent confusion or observable lethargy, especially if repeated—can and does lead to persistent and significant functional and cognitive disabilities.

The National Football League, while still refusing to officially admit to the physical damage caused by head trauma, has instituted a policy that finally goes beyond the medical "Don't Worry Thing" about being "dinged" or "having your bell rung." Anyone experiencing helmet-to-helmet contact and showing any signs of a concussive injury will no longer be allowed to play again for a full week. If there are headaches or any signs of confusion, there will be no playing for two weeks or until all the symptoms have disappeared. Beginning in 2007, there was to be an additional cognitive evaluation that entailed problem-solving and mental nimbleness that the athlete had to pass before being allowed to play again. Football is violent, but then again, so is war.

Everyone agrees to the explosive power of the present day IEDs, yet there is reluctance on the part of the Pentagon, military physicians, and the VA, to entertain the possibility that exposure to these blasts, even dozens of meters from the detonation points, can lead to significant neurological injury and the accompanying functional impairments.

If there is reluctance on the part of the country to understand or be concerned about the dangers as well as the sufferings of those who currently fight our wars, there is an equally a great refusal on the part of the military to acknowledge the damage due to traumatic brain injuries.

These are the soldiers and marines, men and women, who return home from deployments somewhat dazed and a bit forgetful, with headaches and poor balance. Their husbands and wives, fathers and mothers, sometimes wistfully mention to friends and relatives that their returning loved ones never acted like this before, adding simply that they are just not themselves anymore. Those in the Pentagon who refuse to acknowledge these changes as problems, much less as wounds, are caught in another time and in a different place. Reality has left them far behind and they are back to wishful thinking.

The immediate medical issue though, is not whether exposures to IEDs at any distance can cause a TBI, but whether a single or multiple exposures can be the cause of Post Traumatic Stress Disorder. In short, is PTSD a disease of the mind, or is it a disease of the brain? This is not simply an academic issue to the 50,000 troops left in Iraq, or the next 30,000 troops to be sent to Afghanistan. For them it is not merely an interesting or intriquing question, but truly a matter of life and death, pain and suffering. Just ask the family of any returning soldier or marine. Virtually every one of them will have been exposed to an IED at some time during their deployment.

15.

Traumatic Brain Injuries / PTSD / The Invisible Wounds

The real question is whether the so-called mild Traumatic Brain Injuries (mTBIs) cause a lot more damage than we first suspected or were willing to admit. If they are more damaging, then we're back to the shell shock of World War I.

—Conversation: Neurologist, VA hospital

Using numbers alone, one would think there might be a connection between exposures to the concussive effects of an IED and the development of Post Traumatic Stress Disorder. The Rand Corporation has documented that over 300,000 soldiers and marines have been exposed to IEDs, while the Veteran's Administration has calculated that some 320,000 of the troops deployed to Iraq and Afghanistan over the last decade have developed a credible diagnosis of PTSD. It would not be unreasonable to assume that at some level of incidence similar numbers may well mean that the two conditions might be connected or at least be what is now called "co-morbid."

It is not that PTSD has been without its own explanation long before there were high explosives and roadside bombs. History's most famous veteran, Odysseus, upon his return home from the Trojan Wars, looks around and, clearly confused and disoriented, wonders out loud; "Who are these people whose land I have come to…"

Those feelings of Odysseus, of no longer belonging, of reaching home and suddenly being a stranger in a strange land, are shared in some form by virtually every soldier who has been in combat and, upon returning home, is expected to think and act as they did before they were forced to kill or be killed. That much about war has never changed. What we don't know, and what Homer doesn't tell us, is how many times Odysseus might have received blows to the head during his multiple battles in front of the walls of Troy, or on his decade-long adventures as he traveled home.

Fear and terror clearly have their own psychological effects, but so does physical damage to the brain. Schizophrenia, once considered a disease of the mind, is now known to be the result of abnormalities of the chemicals and neuro-transmitters that keep the brain functioning and organized. It is no longer a mental illness where strange voices speak to troubled people, but a medical disease resulting from physically defective transmitters with the ensuing neuronal dysfunctions. No voices, only malformed or misdirected chemicals, a disease of the brain, rather than of the mind.

In this brave new world of high-tech scientific medicine, sorting out the brain from the mind has become, as has all of modern medicine, a matter of accurate weights and even more accurate measurements. The basis of all science may be intuition but the nuts and bolts that hold the sciences together and give science it's credibility are the data points and probability constants. The axiom of science is that "if you can't weigh it or measure it you don't know it." Or put more dramatically, "Forget about the Whys, find out the How." That is certainly now true of psychiatry and psychology, as it is of all of medicine.

The obvious craziness of George the Third, with his black-colored urine, was discovered, in the retrospective microscope of Twenty-first Century medical science, to be the genetically inherited disease porphyria. It is a disease of so-called intermediate metabolism that can damage brain cells by the body's production of abnormal proteins, leading to bizarre and irrational behaviors.

This same sorting out of the body from the mind that happened with schizophrenia happened again in 2010 with the publication in the journal *Science* describing the discovery of a new retrovirus contaminating the nation's blood supply. The virus called XMRV was found in 10 percent of the stored blood. The importance of this finding is that this virus is the same virus that has recently been discovered in over two-thirds of patients with a diagnosis of Chronic Fatigue Syndrome.

Physicians have felt for decades that Chronic Fatigue Syndrome is a psychological and not a medical disorder. Despite considerable effort, no causative agent has ever been found, nor any abnormal bodily function or lab test, to point to a physical cause for the condition. CFS is considered to be a debilitating psychological condition restricted almost entirely to unhappy, upper-middle-class Caucasian women living in the suburbs.

Not only has the XMRV virus been found in a majority of these patients, and not in matched controls without the condition, but there is now a growing concern that contaminated XMRV blood, injected into surgical patients who have experienced significant blood loss, may be the real cause of the ongoing fatigue, exhaustion, and depression that occurs after surgery. It has always been explained away as the stress of the surgical procedure combined with the physical exhaustion of post-operative blood loss.

The scientific article that documented the presence of this virus in patients with Chronic Fatigue Syndrome was titled, "A New Virus for an Old Disease." But scientists did have to find the virus before anyone could connect it to the physical cause of the symptoms. It would appear that the overwhelming exhaustion in these patients, long dismissed as *their* problem and due to the uncontrollable stresses of surgery, may be due to an infection with this newly discovered retrovirus somehow affecting both the body and the brain. A condition that physicians thought, and were able to convince family members, was no more than an indulgent psychological problem turned out to be a real disease caused by a real virus affecting real parts of the body.

Richard Feynman, the famous physicist, would start his graduate level classes on quantum mechanics at Cal Tech by reminding the students that whatever they might think of science, its real value was "that it keeps us from fooling ourselves." What is true of physics is true in medicine. The difficulty in sorting out brain damage from a psychological condition lies in the very complexity of the brain and the need to have very precise tools in order to measure, and document, what is normal, what is not, what has remained healthy, and what is damaged or diseased. And all that starts with the anatomy.

And that is precisely where the issue of TBI and PTSD physically come together.

From the time of the earliest dissections, the brain has been divided on simple observational grounds into gray and white matter, and that is precisely how the brain actually looks. The gray matter is gray because it is made up of layers and layers of densely packed neurons, or brain cells, piled in the hundreds of thousands, one on top of the other, throughout the outer sections of the brain. The white matter, that does indeed look white at surgery or at autopsy, is made up of the axons, long slender microscopic fibers colored white because each individual axon is insulated from all the surrounding axons by a thin outer sheath of a white fatty insulating substance called myelin. It is these covered axons that not only connect the billions of individual neurons within the brain, but eventually come together in ever larger fibrous bundles to form the spinal cord and finally, the large peripheral nerves that carry nervous impulses to the muscles as well as all the different organs of the body. Some of these fibers are only microns in length, while others reaching from the brain to the heart, lungs, kidneys, and the muscles of the arms and legs may be yards long. Electrical signals move up and down these fibers to keep the whole system working together.

The white matter with its billions of axons makes up the wiring of the central nervous system. Some of the largest bundles of these fibers are the axons that connect the neurons of the right side of the brain with the neurons of the left. The largest of these, the Corpus Callosum, lying in the very center of the brain between the brain's two major hemispheres, contains over 200 million fibers. The average internet cable running into your house contains less then 50,000 fibers.

Taken together, the brain is an amazing electrical grid that makes the whole body work, from how we move, to how we see, to why and how our hearts speed up and slow down, to how we continue to breathe in a regular fashion even when we sleep, and why we can think and how we remember. It is no wonder that damage to these fibers leads to all of the problems and symptoms of Multiple Sclerosis. Indeed MS, and other neurological disorders, are classified by neurologists as specific diseases of the brain's white matter that, for some reason, lose their outer protective myelin coating and because of the physical damage to the fibers, can no longer function as designed.

The gray and white matter that make up the major components of the brain, along with the supporting blood vessels and connective tissues, are organized into layers of different densities depending on how many cells, and how many fibers, are packed together into that one specific area of the brain. When examined in a living patient, these different layers of brain tissue have the consistency of differing layers of Jello. It is these different layers of densities that make the brain so exquisitely sensitive to motion, whether from a blow to the head or a passing blast wave from a roadside bomb or suicide bomber.

These different layers of the brain tissues, with their different masses like those different layers of Jello, move at different speeds when set into motion. It is the different speed at which these layers move that generates the internal shearing forces between layers that tear the bridging microscopic veins and arteries, connective tissues, and bridging nerve cells. A brain set in motion is like a layer cake suddenly placed on the top of a jackhammer. And that is happening all the time now in Iraq and in ever increasing numbers in Afghanistan. As the neurosurgeons have pointed out, the damage from that shaking can be more widespread and more neurologically disabling to the person than a brain hit by a bullet.

Shaken Baby Syndrome is the most dramatic example of the damage that can be caused by simply setting a brain into motion. It is well known within pediatrics as a major life-threatening injury of child abuse, leading to significant central nervous system injury including blindness, retardation, and even death. The damage results from the brain moving back and forth within the skull, leading to significant bleeding and damage to the connections between the brain's different layers.

An infant's neck muscles are not strong enough to hold the head steady when the child is being shaken, allowing the head to snap back and forth in rapid succession. The physical forces of the head moving and the brain remaining still are exactly the same as the physical forces that work on a brain moving while the skull remains motionless. In either case, the results are the same. The soft tissues of the frontal and basal lobes of the brain smash up against the rigid inside of the skull, causing significant bruising to the surfaces of the brain, while the inner parts of the brain, moving at different speeds and different distances, tear apart the internal connections.

The dynamics of a shaken baby are basically the same as an adult brain exposed to a helmet-to-helmet shock, hitting the back of your head on the ground while chasing a fly ball, or being exposed to a shock wave from an exploding IED. It is accepted that any or all can lead to physical injury and long-term brain damage, with significant and often cognitive impairment.

There is no trouble in diagnosing the big internal bleeds, the expanding blood clots, or the severe brain swellings, any more than it is difficult to make the diagnosis of a brain tumor or of meningitis. The problem is that the more subtle the injury, the baby that simply hits its head falling to the floor from a chair or the marine standing some distance from an exploding IED, the more difficult to make the diagnosis of a brain injury. You do need some measurement of what is normal and what is not before you can give a diagnosis of injury or damage, that's just how medical diagnosis works.

An adequate determination of mild brain injuries is made even more complicated and confusing by the fact that the most sophisticated imaging techniques of the brain, CT scans and Magnetic Resonance Imaging (MRI), used to diagnose brain damage are best at detecting abnormalities of the gray matter and not precise enough to pick up subtle but real damage to the closely packed bundles of fibers making up the brain's white matter.

The white matter remains the black hole of neurology. In many ways, sorting out damage to the fibers that connect the billions of brain cells is like trying to sort out a problem in the wiring of your computer. With current technology for both your computer and the brain it is difficult at best and in many cases almost impossible. A recent article in the newsletter *Neurology Today* described the medical problem:

> *A patient with a mild traumatic brain injury can pose a challenge to the neurologist—the clinical symptoms may suggest damage within the brain but the CT and MRI are usually normal.*

In layman's terms, a neurologist may have a great deal of clinical information and even suspicion about a potential brain injury, but there is no way to tell whether or not the brain has been structurally damaged if the CT scans and MRIs are read as normal. The open question with major changes in behaviors and alterations in cognitive functions following a potential brain injury is what it has always been, whether there is something wrong with the mind or basically something wrong with the brain.

There is no truly typical head injury. As simple an accident as sitting in a car and being hit from behind and abruptly and unexpectedly slamming your head back into a headrest can do it. For many, this perfectly simple everyday accident, with symptoms of lack of energy, lapses of memory, poor co-ordination, depression, and the "he or she are not themselves anymore," qualifies as a mild Traumatic Brain Injury. These types of injuries, that make up over 85 percent of all brain injuries, are called "mild" because they are maddeningly difficult to confirm based on the fact that all the available brain scans do not display any prominent or focal abnormalities of the brain or surrounding tissues.

The neurologists and neuro-radiologists that see these patients literally have to put down "no significant brain injury" in their reports, making a definitive diagnosis or the ability to obtain damages from insurance companies virtually impossible. But these same physicians and researchers are currently pursuing neuro-chemical and serum markers of brain injury while the brain imaging experts are literally focusing on one of the probable areas of brain injury that up until the present time has been beyond observation or measurement, specifically, Diffuse Axonal Injury or DAI.

Diffuse Axonal Injury is a condition in which head trauma or a shock wave shears the delicate fibers that carry the electrical signals from one brain cell to the next, as well as forming the major nerves that leave the brain, forming the nerves of the spinal column. This type of axonal injury is notorious for eluding all the current imaging, blood, and spinal fluid evaluations, even if the patient is unconscious or severely confused following what has clearly been a head injury. What is clear is that damage to axons can unfold slowly or become worse over days, weeks, and with repeated so-called mTBIs, even over months and years.

It is this gap between symptoms and a definitive diagnosis of axonal injury that has led some psychologists dealing with veterans or active duty personal in Iraq and Afghanistan to a diagnosis of PTSD. By the patient having been exposed to multiple IEDS, or simply having been in a war zone, they recommend an anti-convulsive medication on a trial basis, suspecting the behavioral problems are a result of an mTBI.

If a medication that clearly treats major disruptions of brain function leading to seizures can be of benefit to patients with a diagnosis of PTSD, then one would have to consider a physical change within the brain itself, rather than a psychological diagnosis based on the stresses of the battlefield, even without any official record of history of exposure to a blast wave.

And, as so often happens in today's medicine with its increasing emphasis on technology, there may now be a way to sort out the presence of axonal tears that might lead to a better diagnosis—that at least some of the symptoms of PTSD might indeed be the result of an injury to the brain itself rather than a damaged psyche.

Neuroscience may have finally begun to catch up with the some of the damages, as well as the fears and the heartaches, of going to war. It all began with the clinical observation that there are some characteristics of both concussive injuries and PTSD that are similar, if not identical.

In medicine, whenever you have similar symptoms, you can expect, or have to look for, similar causes. We know from studies of falls and car and motorcycle accidents, that short-term memory loss and poor concentration, irritability and anger, depression, headaches, dizziness, decreased executive functions such as planning or learning a new task, sleep problems, fatigue, and poor balance are all part of what is an mTBI. Even with these symptoms there might be no abnormalities noted on any of the routine imaging techniques. What is troubling is that 30 percent of patients with these symptoms will continue to have the same difficulties a year or more after the injury, indicating what may be both significant and persistent brain damage.

One of the characteristics of military personal with PTSD is poor short-term memory, irritability and anger, episodes of depression and anxiety, as well as fatigue, sleep problems, night-mares, states of hyper-arousal, and intrusive thoughts, including the re-experiencing of the past traumatic events. Clinically many of these symptoms are the same for both diagnoses.

In addition, some 50 percent of civilian patients with what are called "stun injuries" from blows to the head, have the same early and late symptoms as military patients with a diagnosis of PTSD, but these patients are found on CT and MRIs to have bruises of the frontal lobes of the brain.

Yet, the other 50 percent of patients with the same symptoms do not have any changes on the different imaging techniques and neurologists, in the face of the negative CTs and MRIs, have a tendency to call the problem psychological rather than physical. The open question for that 50 percent with stun injuries but normal CTs and MRIs is whether there is something wrong with the brain that has not been noticed on the various brain scans.

We are not supposed, nor are we allowed, to guess anymore in medicine. To have a physical disease you need a physical change. In order to have a diagnosis of strep throat, you do need to have a positive throat culture for Group A Strep. If you have chest pain and are worried about a heart attack, but the angiogram shows open coronary arteries, you are not having a heart attack no matter the pain, even with a strong family history of relatives dying of heart attacks. In a real way, when it comes to the central nervous system, if you can't see an abnormality or measure something that is different from the ordinary or the normal, then there is no organic disease and nothing is said to be physically wrong. That's modern medicine and what patients have to put up with and what physicians are forced to do.

But for the brain at least, that kind of confusion and maybe even nonsense, may finally be coming to an end. If you haven't heard of the Tensor MRI or the more technical term Diffusion Tensor Imaging or (DTI) you will, particularly if you are a soccer-mom or a father with a child playing high school or college football or any of the other sports where there is the possibility of head injuries resulting from helmet-to-helmet impacts.

Diffusion Tensor Imaging is an application of MRI technology that physically measures the direction of movement of individual water molecules throughout the brain's axonal network, or white matter. In intact, undamaged brains the primary direction of movement of the water molecules is parallel to the nerve fibers, giving a precise, well-defined, and well-organized magnetic signal from an undamaged bundle of fibers. But when neuronal axons, even individual nerve fibers, are damaged, the movement of the water molecules throughout and along the fiber is disrupted, the molecules become less aligned even without any of the other usual signs of nerve damage, including bleeding or swellings. A change in the Tensor MRIs signal indicates damage, or at least some kind of physical disruption, along individual axons or within bundles of nerve fibers at that precise anatomical point of the signal shift.

Recently a pediatric neurologist in the Department of Clinical Neuroscience at the University of Minnesota gave a lecture, "Mild Traumatic Brain Injury: What is the role of Brain Imaging, such as Diffusion Tensor Imaging, in the Evaluation of these Patients?" The objective of this lecture for the assembled physicians was to understand the value of this new brain imaging technique in the evaluation of a possible mTBI.

The take-home lesson was that if you are a parent and your child hits his or her head and is the least bit confused or disoriented or later has headaches or simply "isn't themselves," but otherwise looks and acts quite normal, you still want to see a physician and you might want to obtain a Diffusion Tensor MRI. You would certainly want to have the imaging test if there were any ongoing neurological or cognitive issues.

The Tensor MRI, unlike routine MRIs and CT scans, is exquisitely sensitive down below the cellular levels to any physical changes within the tiniest fibers of the white matter. Diffusion Tensor Imaging fills in the gap of brain damage investigation, that of evaluating the fibers that make up the brain's circuitry. With a Tensor MRI, all of the brain can be adequately, equally, and definitively imaged, gray and white matter alike.

The experimental use of this new technique has demonstrated that conventional MR imaging underestimates the extent of axonal injury following even a mild TBI. With a new test, there are always new medical insights and new clinical understandings and the beginning use of the Tensor MRI is proving no different.

A recent study published in the *American Journal of Neuropathology* proves that fact. The radiologists using a Tensor MRI evaluated the brains of a group of patients with a diagnosis of mTBIs with persistent post-concussive symptoms determined by the use of the standard head injury checklist that included the presence of headaches, fatigue, dizziness, irritability, anxiety or depression, difficulty sleeping, and personality changes or apathy, as entrance into the study. Exclusion criteria included any history of neurological or psychiatric illness including drug or alcohol abuse.

Conventional MRI and CT scans had been read as normal in all the patients. But with the Tensor MRI, half of the patients who showed no bleeding clearly had obvious damage to their brain's white matter. The article ended with this warning:

Patient reports of a post-concussion syndrome (including what neuropsychologists call the higher executive functions that allow for planning for future events) may be dismissed in the context of normal findings on CT or conventional MR Imaging. These studies indicate axonal shear injury to be the primary mechanism of (brain) damage in mild TBIs.

It seems that the Tensor MRIs are uniquely suited to detect significant microscopic white matter injuries, and just in time. With the sending of troops to Afghanistan, where they are sure to be exposed to more numerous and ever more powerful IEDs, there is sure to be more evidence of brain damage, along with significantly more symptoms of PTSD. Is it cause and effect, or merely an association? On our newest battlefields, that may well be a distinction without a difference.

Yet neither the Congress, a body rarely known for foresight that has never adequately funded the medical needs of our soldiers and marines, nor the last or current administration, nor the Pentagon or VA, has ordered or purchased a single Tensor MRI, which is basically a very sophisticated computer program running on an MRI platform. The hundreds of medical facilities along the evac-chain and all of the stateside hospitals will have to function without this technology to counter the new type of injuries suffered by the troops in the new type of warfare.

It might also be that a diagnosis of a TBI rather than PTSD may, by definition, result in a life-long service-connected disability claim to be paid to each disabled veteran for the rest of his or her life. VA Disability Claims, like Social Security and Medicare, are entitlements, and by law, entitlements once in place last for the lifetime of the recipient. PTSD, for all of its anguish, is considered a treatable psychological condition and so the liability of the VA, and the government, is limited to approved and time-limited treatment periods, with an expectation of ultimate success within relatively short periods of time. No need for long-term or life-time disability claims.

But that may just be the cynic's view. Still, it is a view based on what occurred during the Vietnam War, when thousands of veterans were denied life-time claims after receiving a diagnosis of PTSD. It may also be the reason that the economists Linda Bilmes and Joseph Stiglitz have put the national costs for Iraq and Afghanistan at over 3 trillion dollars without PTSD becoming an entitlement.

And that number of 3 trillion dollars is if every one of our soldiers and marines went home today and there were no new deaths and no new injuries.

It is not that those running the military today don't understand what is going on. The Chief of Staff of the Medical Corps for the Army, when asked in a recent interview on National Public Radio if TBIs had become the signature wounds of Afghanistan and Iraq, gave a qualified yes, admitting that based on the military's own data from their Wounded Warriors Program, PTSD had to be considered the real signature wound of the wars, with 45 percent of those in the program being diagnosed with PTSD, followed by 17 percent with TBIs, and 12 percent with amputations.

When pushed, the general admitted that if PTSD were shown to be the result of TBIs, then brain injuries would clearly have to be these wars' signature injury. What the general did not address was the distinct possibility that a TBI of any severity might well make the soldier or marine more susceptible to PTSD. In short, that one may make the soldier or marine more susceptible to the other. And that is the growing concern among the psychiatrists in the Department of Defense hospital system, as well as the physicians and psychologists in the VA's poly-trauma and mental health units.

The general did admit that poor record-keeping in both Iraq and Afghanistan regarding who was exposed to an IED may indeed make these connections impossible. If there is nothing in the records, or those records are not available during or after deployments, then changing a diagnosis of PTSD to a mild TBI becomes impossible, whatever the symptoms.

So why not just do what some within the military do and VA systems are beginning to advocate? Simply being in a combat zone is to be exposed to an IED and goes on the record.

But in the end that may simply add to the 3 trillion dollars that these wars have already cost. And apparently that is not something this Congress or this administration is willing to do.

What is clear is that additional funding for research is needed to be able to distinguish PTSD from mTBIs. We certainly need the government to order a few Tensor MRIs. We owe that much to the few we have sent to do so much for all the rest of us.

16.

ALL THE JAKES / ADRIFT IN AFGHANISTAN / 2010

The Korangal Valley is sort of the Afghanistan of Afghanistan: too remote to conquer, too poor to intimidate, too autonomous to buy off.
— Sebastian Junger, *War*

Since the end of the Civil War, we have had a Southern army. The majority of our company and general grade officers, as well as high-level NCOs come from southern cities and towns of less than 7,000 people. That's not so bad. If you want leaders who understand the real meaning of victory, ask the ones who have been defeated.

But then again, the South might just be different. In many ways, it has never been "the United States *is*" so much as "the United States *are.*" And the South is part of that "*are.*" Nobody up North, out West, or in the East talks about being able to kill "your own snakes" or ever uses the words "splendid behavior" to talk about someone's actions. I learned how to drink whiskey in the Army. There was not a single company grade officer or senior NCO I met during my two years on active duty in the military, or those decades afterwards of keeping up with old army friends while making new ones, who drank Scotch or bourbon. It is Old Grand Dad, Early Times, Wild Turkey, and Southern Comfort. Not so bad.

Yet despite the obvious difference in drinking habits, for many from the South it is all still Gettysburg and Antietam, Spotsylvania and the Battle of the Wilderness. These officers and NCOs from below the Mason-Dixon line like to win, but they hate losing even more. And that must have been something that Jake picked up.

It wasn't that Jake had not seen pictures of relatives in their uniforms all his life, but seeing is not necessarily believing. Still, he did look at the pictures on the walls of his parents' home out in the hallways and going up the steps to the bedrooms for as long as he could remember. There was that sense of serving in the very air of the house, even though no one still alive ever talked about their time in the military and definitely never mentioned, even in passing, about having been in combat.

David Haberstram, the *New York Times* reporter in Vietnam and the author of *The Making of a Quagmire,* published in 1969 about the growing disaster unfolding in Vietnam, and seven years later, *The Best and the Brightest,* documenting the disaster that had indeed become Vietnam, explained that as a child in New York City in the late 1940s, he'd go out into the courtyards of the apartment buildings and watched his uncles and their friends, all veterans of the Second World War, play pick-up basketball after work or on their way back and forth from college paid for by the GI Bill.

They'd play shirts and skins. He remembered sitting on the steps of the fire escapes, startled and amazed that everyone who played skins had a scar, a part of a muscle or a limb gone, a bone that was clearly missing, or a strange limp when they ran.

The stunning part to the young Halberstam was that it was everybody. No one had escaped. No one had been spared. But no one ever said a word. No one offered an explanation for their wound or their infirmity, nor was anyone ever asked for or expected to give one. According to Halberstam, no one mentioned the war. No one complained or appeared offended or even troubled by the wounds. No one asked for help or to slow things down. And no one offered up an excuse, even if they tripped when they ran or couldn't quite handle the ball as well as they should have. They were just there to play basketball. It was only much later in Vietnam that Halberstam was to realize that these were the ones who had survived.

In a very real way, watching those shirts and skins pick-up games, the young future reporter had caught the essence of combat. Everyone was at risk and what finally happened was simply a matter of chance or luck. That was what was so scary and so real and why everyone kept so silent about combat. No one talked about it and no one asked why half the muscles of a shoulder or along the neck were gone. They already knew. They didn't have to ask.

Jake was not only raised in the quiet shadows of the military, but in the shadow of the Marines. Jake's mother's twin brother had been in the Marines. Two of her other brothers were in the Army. Jake's father's younger sister had been in the Army in the '80s and his brother in the Marines. His father, too, had been in the Marines when the Marine barracks in Beirut had been blown up. There were two grandfathers, one who had been a captain of a frigate during the Korean War, and the other who fought in the Army throughout the whole of the Second World War in Italy and Germany.

Much like Halberstam was drawn to the silence of those wounded and crippled veterans playing basketball in the alleys of New York City, Jake had been drawn to the very silence of those pictures. Toward the end of Jake's senior year in high school, his father, concerned about his son's two older friends who had already graduated and not gone to college and were without jobs and just lying around all day, was determined that his son would not end up the same way. So he sat Jake down one Sunday and gave him three options after graduation: college, working full time, or the military.

Jake didn't argue or, for that matter, even have to think about it. Later, his father would remember how simple it had been and how matter-of-fact. "That's OK," Jake said, "I don't think I have the grades for a really good college. I'm going to enlist." It was almost as if his son had grown up right there in front of him, even as they were talking.

175

That was March 2007. The war in Iraq was not going well. In fact, the whole country was approaching the abyss. Iraq had descended into a full-scale civil war, with 1,000 civilians dying each month. The gunmen of Al Qaeda, along with their suicide bombers, were carrying out large-scale massacres of Shiite civilians, and the Shiite militias, some in Iraqi Army uniforms and supported by Iran, retaliated by massacring thousands of young Sunni men. Iraq seemed lost, with American troops hopelessly caught up in the turmoil and being killed and wounded in increasing numbers by both sides.

None of this was of any real concern to Jake. He was right about not having the grades to get into a first-rate college and everyone, including his father, knew that an entrance-level job would have bored him, while still giving him plenty of time to goof off and get into trouble.

So Jake and his father went down to the recruiting offices inside the Air National Guard Terminal at the Metropolitan Airport. Jake kept his preference to himself as to which branch of the armed services he was considering.

The Navy was out from the beginning. Jake had no desire to go to war on a ship and had no interest in flying off aircraft carriers. The Army recruiter was almost too slick about the benefits of service, including bonus pay and the fact that having military experience would be a plus for any future civilian employment.

The Marine recruiter offered nothing except being the point of the spear. "The first in. And the last out." Jake's father went along because he thought that with his being there and being a veteran that none of the recruiters would go off the deep end or run the risk of lying. But he did feel that the Marine recruiter had offered more of the truth than any of the other recruiters. Jake saw that too and with his father having been in the Marines, made that same choice.

"It's the Marines," he said. Walking back to the car, his whole demeanor changed. They had gone to the recruiting offices as father and son, and had left as two marines. As they approached the car, Jake stopped. "If it's all right with you," he said, "I'd like to enlist right away. At least as soon as the paper work is ready. There's no sense waiting."

Jake went back on his own to the recruiting office early the next week. He called his parents to tell them that if they wanted to watch him sworn in that they should drive out to the recruiting center, that he'd wait until they got there. His mother managed to be proud.

Jake's parents laid off him for those last few months of school, letting Jake do pretty much what he wanted. Iraq was still out there. But the surge was working. By degrading Al-Qaeda's leadership, the influx of new troops was able to reduce the scope of the civil war. This allowed everyone to take a deep breath and step back from what had been an approaching catastrophe.

Afghanistan was back in the news. The Marines, who wanted no part of garrison duty and baby-sitting any kind of new Iraqi nation-building, had put Afghanistan back up on their front burner and were lobbying the Pentagon to send them to Helmand Province.

The surge had bought us time in Iraq to try to buy us time in Afghanistan. It might well have been the time for counter-insurgency rather than counter-terrorism, but even with counter-insurgency, you still have to kill the bad guys.

Jake took his parents up on their obvious lack of supervision during those last few months of school. But the two wars and the Marines were always out there, like a worrisome breeze blowing in from the future. The day after graduation, Jake said that it made no sense to wait until the end of September, which was his enlistment date. He had the date pushed up and went into the Marines on July 12, 2008.

It was the week that a unit of the 173rd Airborne Brigade occupying the Wanat Outpost in the Konregal Valley in Eastern Afghanistan was attacked by over 200 Taliban. The battle, described by those who were there as the " Blackhawk Down" of the Afghanistan War, went on for almost half the day. The firefights in Iraq usually lasted no more than half an hour.

The forty-eight Americans and seventy-four Afghan soldiers were outnumbered three to one. At the end of the battle, nine

U.S. troops were dead and twenty-seven were wounded, a casualty rate of 80 percent. The 245-page After Action Report describes the fight "as remarkable as any small unit action in American military history," including those in Vietnam. The report, created by a member of the Army's Combat Study Institute at Fort Leavenworth, Kansas, details automatic weapons that turned white-hot and jammed from non-stop firing, while the severely wounded continued to feed ammunition to those still able to use their weapons. The battle ended only when helicopter gunships and F-15s strafed and bombed the Taliban positions, killing dozens of the attackers.

The AAR cited a lack of preparation time for the 173rd before being sent from Iraq to Afghanistan. The strong implication that fighting on the desert plains of Iraq within an urban population, with well-developed roads and other types of substantial infrastructure, was different, and should have been recognized as different, than fighting village tribesmen in isolated valleys and mountain areas.

There were also tactical concerns about the total absence of an operational plan for the combat that was sure to lie ahead for the 173rd. After all, the Russians had fought in those same mountains for more than a decade and were never able to occupy or control any of the major mountain passes or valleys. And the Russians had a force of over 250,000 troops with absolutely no rules of engagement—able to kill and blow up anyone and anything they wanted.

But the real explanation for the failure at Wanat was centered on the fact that the U.S. forces had faced off against a far more sophisticated enemy than they had faced in Iraq or in Afghanistan in 2001. The world of fighting in Afghanistan had changed in the eight years we'd been there and apparently nobody in charge had noticed.

The report stated that, "The Taliban can and does now operate as a disciplined armed force, using well-rehearsed small unit tactics that can challenge the American military for dominance on the conventional battlefield."

There were other lessons that should have been learned in our seven years in both Iraq and Afghanistan. The areas that had been chosen for our outposts were linked by rutted trails easily blocked and sabotaged, while Wanat itself could only be reached quickly by helicopter.

Those at Wanat never had the construction equipment to build adequate fortifications for, as the report explains, a "defensible outpost," while a lack of fresh water and currency to buy favors and win the support of the villagers surrounding the outpost had been contributing factors to the lack of military preparedness.

More importantly, there was a lack of an increase in air surveillance once the commanders had made the mistake of attending a village council uninvited. It made clear, to anyone who understood the local customs, that the Americans were not welcomed there.

The numbers of killed and wounded civilians from air strikes over the preceding eight years had added an element of revenge to the centuries-old dislike of any foreigners. There is an Afghan expression that has not changed in some 3,000 years: "You might decide whether or not you come into our valley, but we will decide if we let you out."

At times during the daylong battle of Wanat, there were sustained individual firefights at distances of less than ten meters. During the later part of the battle, Taliban fighters managed to work their way through the concertina wire that was the only defense against an attack, killing the platoon commander with a volley of AK-47 rounds. The morning after the battle, what remained of the 173rd was pulled out of Wanat. The outpost was simply abandoned.

For those who remembered, it was all eerily similar to "Hamburger Hill" in Vietnam. The 101st Airborne fought the North Vietnamese to a standstill, suffering more than 500 casualties, only to pack up and go back to their base camp the next day, giving whatever it was that they'd been fighting for back to whomever had held the mountain the day before the battle began. There is some thought now, as part of the surge in Afghanistan and for tactical reasons, of sending the Marines back to Wanat, though whatever unit they send back will not have an easy time of it.

The Marines though, did learn something about how to fight in Iraq, and have begun to use that learning as they have been shifted to the mountains and plains of Afghanistan. In war, as in education, it is never what you teach, so much as what you emphasize, that is important.

The Marine lobbying had paid off and units were moved out of Iraq into Helmand Province to re-supply U.S. bases that had already been there. The Marines understand that while you might have to show a friendly and helpful face, someone is still going to have to do the fighting and in Afghanistan those fights would be difficult and deadly. That whole "First in and Last out" hasn't changed in some 250 years. But as Jake's father had learned, and now Jake was to find out, neither had basic training.

Basic training for the Marines has remained what it has always been. It is the "tear you down and then build you up again" process, only this time as a marine. Whatever else might be said of the Marines, they are not very good at mending fences and would rather be respected or feared than liked.

For Jake, it was not so much that a new person emerged, but rather that the Jake who had always been there gradually took over. Still, there are very few eighteen-year-olds who will not grow up a little by learning that, when someone tells you to do something, they expect you to do it. Life is supposed to be, and usually is, a very serious and demanding place. That in itself could become the Marine's motto.

Jake took his thirteen weeks of basic training at the Marine Corps Recruit Depot in San Diego. He didn't feel the training was as difficult, or as trying, as his father had warned. There had been some tough moments though, when sleep-deprived and exhausted, he barely managed to keep going; a few times, he almost didn't. But in the Marines, "almost" doesn't count. If you do it, you do it. In the world of the Marines, the real things are sometimes just that simple.

But even with that, Jake felt that things had been turned down a notch to get everyone through the thirteen weeks. In a way he was right. Some Marine units had already been deployed five or six times to Iraq. The Corps was feeling the strain and needed all the men and women they could get, even if they weren't quite ready yet.

Everyone in Jake's class—with the edge taken off of the most difficult parts of the training—made it through Basic, though there were a few that he wasn't so sure would be there if things went wrong. What he did learn from the Drill Instructors, what all of them learned, was that if you don't fight back you are doomed. The assumptions they'd all grown up with, that if you were nice to people, they would be nice to you, was a lie, and that the best response to force was force, a preparation for the moment, maybe months away, when people they didn't even know would be trying to kill them. It was sobering, and he understood that is was realistic. It was an attitude, if not yet an understanding, that would soon save his life and the lives of others around him. In the end, Marines break things and kill people or they die.

From Basic Training, Jake went on to Marine Combat Training at Camp Pendleton. It was deadly and impressive. The Marines had never believed the message of "Mission Accomplished." Since the invasion of Iraq, the training had grown more focused and more intense. Whatever else was going to happen in Iraq, the enemy would have to have more than good planning or luck to kill a bunch of Marines. Jake told his father with absolute confidence during one of his phone calls home that no one could stand up to a 50-caliber machine gun. "You can't even hide from one."

Jake's father heard the respect and awe in the very calmness of his son's voice. Whatever else was might be happening, his son was growing up. In Afghanistan, the 50 was to become Jake's favorite weapon. It would be the weapon that would save his life and the lives of those around him.

At the end of MCT, Jake received an MOS as an Audio Communication Specialist and went on with a small group of trainees to the Marine base at Twenty-nine Palms, California for six weeks of training as a field radio operator, ending up with an "0261" or MOS of Field Radio Operator.

After Basic and MCT, the six weeks at Twenty-nine Palms weren't all that hard. It was mostly classroom work and Jake became a gym rat. Somehow he knew that being in shape was as much a part of being a marine as was the whole issue of survival and being able to use a weapon better then your enemy. He didn't want to have to blame himself if things went bad or went wrong. Besides, they had gone far enough in their training to begin hearing stories about Afghanistan from those who'd been there and had managed to make it back home.

These weren't quite cautionary tales, but reality stories of having to carry fifty pounds of body armor at times moving straight up, while the bad guys wearing sandals and carrying some water and an RPG or AK-47 with a dozen rounds of ammunition, jumped from rock to rock like billy goats.

Following Communications School, Jake slimmed down and buffed out. He went back to Pendleton not only unable to fit into the T-shirts he'd been issued the first day of Basic, but having to find pants two sizes smaller at the waist. He learned how to communicate with most of the world at the same time that he'd become able to protect himself and defend the nation.

He took the communications training very seriously. A First Sergeant told him at the very beginning of his training that in a battle or a firefight, the radio is going to be yours and your unit's most important weapon.

"You call in what you need—artillery, gunships, fighter-bombers, reinforcements, med-evacs. Without the radio, you may not be killed but you will be fucked." Jake was ready to be a Marine and not just act like one.

At Pendleton, he was assigned to the 1/5 (1st Battalion, 5th Marine Regiment, 1st Marine Division). The day he received his unit patch, a helicopter flying through the Kunar Valley in Helmand Province, ferrying a reduced company of Marines to an outpost near the Kaligal River, was shot down. It was the exact same spot where, twenty years before, Russian helicopters were shot down ferrying Russian troops into that same river basin. It was close to the bridge destroyed 2,300 years earlier by Afghan tribesmen who had trapped half of Alexander the Great's Army, forcing him to marry the daughter of the local tribal chieftain to get what was left of his troops out of Afghanistan and into India.

A week into Pendleton, the newly regrouped and outfitted 1/5 went back to Twenty-nine Palms to spend a month at Mojave Viper, an exact replica of an Afghan village set out in the desert. Those marines already in Iraq were being sent to Helmand Province in Afghanistan, along with the new deployments from the States.

Jake thought the four weeks at the village was useful. It certainly seemed real enough, but there was way too much lecture stuff. You didn't have to spend a whole afternoon in a classroom doing diversity training to figure out that Muslim villagers still living in pre-biblical times had different views on common courtesy and how women should be treated. You could also be pretty sure that a villager of any age or sex might not like Christian soldiers walking around behind sunglasses, armed to the teeth, looking for all the world like Imperial Storm Troopers out of Star Wars—even if they were handing out candy and offering to build better roads and new schools.

The 1/5 left for Afghanistan on May 28, 2009. Jake called his parents to say good-by and tell them not to worry. Jake's father managed to wish him good luck without his voice cracking. His mother didn't do so well.

The 5,000 marines of the 1/5 flew into Manas Airbase in Kyrgyzstan and from there to Bagram Airbase near Kabul. They were put into trucks and taken to Camp Leatherneck, the large Marine base in Helmand Province. From there, the 1,300 Marines in Jake's headquarters supply company moved out to their operational area some eighty miles north of Camp Leatherneck.

Despite the 110-degree heat, they wore full body armor, their M-4's locked and loaded as they took off in their armored Humvees, armored personnel carriers, and MRAPs for the Forward Operating Base (FOB) Geronimo in the Grit Valley, a supply route into Helmand Province and eventually the city of Kandahar. They were to protect the supply convoys to and out of Geronimo. No marines had been in the area since the war had shifted to Iraq in 2003.

The week before Jake's unit had left for Geronimo, the Taliban in Pakistan had blown up a major bridge leading into Afghanistan. They then systematically destroyed a convoy of some forty stranded tankers that were carrying gasoline and aviation fuel to the military bases in Western Afghanistan, including their FOB in the Grit Valley. They'd be short of fuel for a month once they got to Geronimo.

Jake looked at the map of Helmand Province at Camp Leatherneck and figured that his company would be covering an area of a couple of hundred square miles—until someone told him that Helmand Province itself was over 78,000 square miles. Looking again at the map, Jake was surprised to find that Afghanistan was literally twice the size of Iraq and apparently had 10 million more people. And as far as he could tell, there weren't more than three cities in the whole country.

There was a legend on one of the maps that stated there were more than 45,000 villages scattered across the country and up into the mountains bordering Pakistan. It didn't take a genius to realize that 13,000 troops, 50,000, or even half a million, could easily get lost here. What Jake didn't know was that others looking at similar maps through all the centuries had much the same feelings.

When it became clear to the Russian generals that they were failing in Afghanistan, they recommended that the majority of the Russian Army, some 5 million troops, be sent there. The Soviet Government, realizing the foolishness of that recommendation, simply said no. Three years later the Russians were gone, having left for home. But it wasn't only the Russians. After the whole British Expeditionary Force of over 20,000 men were killed in Afghanistan in 1842, Kipling wrote these lines: "If you find yourself wounded on the Afghan Plains and the women come out to cut up what remains; then roll to your rifle and blow out your brains and go to your Gawd like a soldier." It was neither irony nor poetic license. It was the truth.

If Jake felt alone on those first few supply convoys, he understood that the marines out in the villages in platoon-sized outposts were in a worse situation. If they were attacked, it would be life or death from the first shot. The only way to survive out there would be for the villagers to help, or at least warn the different garrisons about an impending attack. Without warning or constant overhead air surveillance, the Taliban could be on top of you before you knew it.

At least at Geronimo, they'd had the equipment to bulldoze the dunes around the base into a reasonably effective barrier. All they took as incoming was the occasional mortar round or some poorly directed sniper fire. Jake's orders took his company, their trucks, his Humvee, his radio command net, and his 50-caliber machine gun out over the most dangerous roads, river basins, and plains in the world.

It was terribly hot, during the middle of the day upwards of 120 degrees, and dusty, the kind of dust that got into your mouth, your food, all the equipment, wheel hubs, and gear trains. For weeks, no Taliban were seen.

But in the mountains, it was different.

The marines up there were always being ambushed. There were almost daily probing movements around the perimeters of their outposts. Some of the mountain areas were almost impassible. It was all straight up and straight down with sixty pounds of gear on your back, and you couldn't see very far and you couldn't see very much.

The Taliban had time to organize a battle plan, stockpile weapons and ammunitions, and attack the bases and outposts where and when they wanted. The mountains also made the use of helicopters and fighter-bombers problematical. The helicopters didn't work well above nine or ten thousand feet, the air is too thin at those heights for good lift and in the hot weather with the hot air rising, even less so. You couldn't get med-evacs in, so at times the marines would have to carry the wounded down off the mountains on stretchers. Even with their own medics, they lost a number of wounded by not getting the right care during that golden hour after being hit.

But it wasn't only the thin air, the Taliban could easily shoot down gunships in the narrow passes leading to the valleys. Any chopper flying into and out of the valleys would have to come dangerously close to the sheer cliffs of the canyon walls. It was the perfect place to bring down a chopper that could not maneuver and had to take only one path in or out through the mountains.

The need for re-supply, as well as the widely scattered and difficult-to-defend outposts, left marines everywhere scrambling just to hang on. With the choppers always flying out at the edge of their "specks" and the danger of being shot down in the steep mountains and narrow canyons always a concern, most of the supplies had to come in by road.

And that was a problem where the roads were easily sabotaged. Supplying 30,000 troops by trucks on roads coming in from Pakistan was already a problem. Jake heard that some of the marines in the mountains had run out of ammunition, while others, who had to keep firing during what were prolonged firefights, had burned out one M-4 barrel after another until they'd run out of barrels.

But in the wide expanses of Helmand Province, it was IEDs. Around Geronimo, the Taliban didn't have to show and run the risk of being killed by attack helicopters or bombing runs of the fighter planes. They could plant the IEDs without being seen, or pay villagers to do it for them.

The open plains of Helmand Province, along with the hundreds of miles of deserts and dry riverbeds, gave everyone a wide view of the surroundings. They could plant their IEDs, be able to see where you were from a distance, and set off the explosives at just the right time to do the most damage and kill the most marines.

As far as Jake could see, for the 1/5 and the convoys they guarded, as well as the marines in the different outposts, winning simply meant surviving. He remembered how back at Camp

186

Leatherneck, some sergeants mumbling that the only way they'd be able to pull this off was to have a lot more troops on the ground.

The immediate problem the 1/5 faced were the roadside bombs, which could be buried anywhere. There were no paved roads, so planting an IED meant simply digging a hole and putting in the explosives with a detonator plate, or hooking it up to some detonator cord that you cover with dirt and set off from half a mile away.

Holes and ruts on the roads were everywhere. It was impossible to tell what was recently dug. Even in the short time that Jake was there, the Taliban had begun using more powerful bombs and were clearly becoming more sophisticated in their use. It didn't seem to matter to them if it was armored vehicles or foot patrols. They were out to simply kill Americans.

The book *The Good Soldiers* describes exactly how it happens and it happened all the time.

"They drove with headlights off and night-vision goggles on that at 12:35 a.m. flared into blindness. Here came the explosion. It came through the doors ... it was perfectly aimed and perfectly timed, and now one of the soldiers was on fire..."

When they'd first arrived in Helmand Province, the Taliban had set the IEDs to explode when a vehicle passed over the pressure plate. When they started to use rollers out in front of the armored vehicles to set off the explosives, the Taliban reset the plates with a time delay so that the explosive charge would not go off under the rollers, but under the vehicle.

The explosive charges were themselves becoming more sophisticated and more powerful. Jake had seen 40-ton MRAPs turned over, with everyone inside having either broken bones or head injuries. As for the foot patrols, if the Taliban spaced the charges just right, with a good view of the path the Marines were taking, and judged their distances correctly, they were sure to kill or wound everyone in that squad and most likely cause a concussion in everyone, if it were a platoon.

A large IED took out one of their armored vehicles during a convoy patrol. Everyone inside except the gunner and the driver were killed. The chopper on the med-evac was shot down coming in to take out the wounded. Jake could swear that he had seen the smoke trail of a rocket coming out of the hills near them a moment before the chopper exploded. It was amazing, but even without the med-evac their medic managed to keep the two alive, having to do a tracheotomy on the gunner right there on the side of the road.

The medic had wrestled the gunner quiet. While the rest of them set up a perimeter defense, he took out his knife and, grabbing the protruding piece of jaw bone, forced back the soldier's head and calmly cut open his throat, then punched a hole into the windpipe. A sputtering of blood and foam came out through the incision, and as his breathing eased, the marine quickly quieted. There was another explosion up ahead and the rattling of small-arms fire. Jake watched while the medic took an endotracheal tube out of his kit, slipped it in through the incision, and threaded it down into the soldier's lungs, listening for the normal inward and outward hiss of air, then reached for the morphine.

They managed to carry both of the wounded down to a Humvee, jury-rigged to carry the stretchers. They would try to make it back to their base camp. It had gotten to the point in their area of operation that if you could hear the boom, it was good. It meant that you were still alive after the bomb went off. A number of those who were near an IED when it went off would be confused and rattled after the explosion even if there were no obvious wounds. But they would tell everyone that they were fine and just walk away to go back to what they were doing.

Jake's war soon had nothing to do with winning hearts and minds, protecting the civilian population, and not shooting up wedding parties, but simply making it back to base camp with the job done, the supplies delivered, and all the equipment intact, with nobody killed or severely wounded. That was called a good day.

There had been a U.S. Aid project during the 1950s in some of the areas they were patrolling. Engineers had dug canals through the valley to bring water to the crops of wheat and corn. Now, the crops were opium poppies and marijuana, with some of the plants five and six feet high. In some places the crops were so dense that is was almost impossible to walk through the fields. When the crops were planted to the edge of the roads, the fields were perfect places for ambushes, which the Taliban could not resist. In Helmand Province that could be a big mistake. Every now and then, the Taliban would do something that foolish.

One early morning, the marines took some fire from the edge of a poppy field. Jake was on top of his APC, manning the 50-cal. He used the machine gun to mow down the plants as surely as if he were using a scythe. They killed ten Taliban that morning and had no more trouble on that part of the road for weeks. The marines always preferred a straight-up firefight to what they called the "death at every corner" crawl that they had used in Iraq and in the larger towns and villages of Afghanistan.

During his months at Geronimo, Jake spared his parents the worst of it. He didn't mention the time that his 50-caliber and two others on accompanying Humvees, along with their Mark 19 automatic grenade launchers, stopped a column of supply trucks and oil tankers from being blown up and all the drivers killed or taken prisoner.

Jake stayed on the top of his Humvee out in the open, bullets ricocheting off the armored plates surrounding him, his own machine gun chewing up the surrounding hillsides, keeping the Taliban from moving closer. After gunships were called in, the Taliban, hearing the sounds of the approaching helicopters, had no choice but to leave or be killed.

While at Geronimo Jake had heard about a shift in strategy to counter-insurgency, whatever that was. When someone asked a sergeant what that meant, the sergeant, clearly annoyed, shrugged it off, muttering that counter-insurgency only came in two sizes—long and very long.

Moving around as much as they did, Jake saw that things weren't going as well as the official pronouncements. There was a lot that wasn't going right. But it was the kids that troubled him the most.

When the 1/5 had first gotten to Helmand Province, the kids would be cheerful and jabbered whenever they stopped or pulled over to wait or rest for a while. They passed out candy and kids would take it. But as the weeks past, the villagers seemed to be keeping their kids away from them. Those who did come up weren't smiling as they did previously, some of the older kids had actually taken to throwing rocks at them when they passed through the villages.

The Taliban might have become more cautious in trying to stick them in the eye, but they were obviously warning the villagers not to help. And Jake couldn't blame villagers for listening. Over the years, the plains had been swept by U.S. and NATO troops countless numbers of times. After a couple of weeks, the troops would just get up and leave and the Afghans who'd helped, or been given work, were worse off. There were stories that Jake believed were true about the Taliban coming back into a village after the American or NATO troops had left and killing all the men who had worked for them, even killing the kids who had acted as lookouts for the American or NATO troops.

Jake understood that if things didn't change, really change, that they'd probably have to leave like everyone else. The Afghan Government knew it. The Afghan people knew it, and the Taliban knew it. And that didn't make much sense to him as they crawled slowly along another dirt road, always looking for signs of recent digging—places where the Marines weren't quite liked anymore, and definitely were not trusted.

There were rumors about new orders coming down from Central Command changing the Rules of Engagement. Apparently, the higher ups were growing more concerned about the increasing numbers of civilian casualties, and to cut down on the collateral damage they were changing the rules to shoot only at people who were shooting at you. But Jake had no idea how to tell the good guys from the bad guys before they actually started shooting. It would be like walking down one of the streets at home, trying to decide whether the person coming towards you was Catholic or Lutheran. If you had to wait for someone to be shooting at you before you could fire back, you'd probably be dead even before you could pull the trigger. To do something like this was lunacy.

Jake heard an officer comment one evening that this fight was not about the Taliban, nationalism, or terrorism, but what he called "valleyism." Jake didn't say anything. He just listened, but reluctantly had to agree. These people only care about what is happening in their own valley. These Afghans have never known any central government and they'd never liked or tolerated any occupying force, whoever they were. He just couldn't see how what they were doing would work. Whatever else was going on or whatever else people were being told, Afghanistan was not going to be easy.

There were comments from the British troops who were still in Afghanistan as part of the shrinking NATO coalition that, whatever they did or however successful the American offensive might appear to be, the fighting would be dropping off during the fall months no matter what happened. "As soon as the leaves start falling off the trees," the Brits offered, "the Afghans fighters give up and go home, since they can be seen more easily maneuvering with the leaves gone. During winter nobody can fight, so the only way you'll be able to tell if you are actually winning is to wait for the spring and see if the fighting starts up again at the same level that it ended. That's the way it's been here for the last 3,000 years. Nothing is going to change just because you guys are here with your gunships and armored personnel carriers. After all," they would add with British understatement, "this is Afghanistan."

Jake did guard duty when one of the captains went out to speak with a group of elders in one of the valleys. It was crazy. The captain talked about putting a paved road through the valley. It would allow the locals to make more money, to make them richer. But what the captain wanted was to have them help the Marines with security. If they did that, then the captain would bring all kinds of money and projects to the valley. Jake doubted that would ever happen and was put off that bringing lots of money to the valley was the reason they were there and getting killed.

Like all nineteen-year-olds, Jake was into music and an avid listener of tapes and disks from rap to country and western, including the oldies but goodies. There were days coming back from patrols that he couldn't help but wonder if the new Twenty-first Century Creedence Clearwater version of "Waist Deep in the Muddy" that ended with "It will be a long dark night before this thing is done" didn't say it better, and maybe more sadly, for his war than Pete Seeger had said it for Vietnam.

A week after the meeting with the elders, Jake heard that six U.S. advisors had been killed at an Afghan National Police Training Center near Kandahar. Apparently, a trainee had turned around at one of the rifle ranges and shot the six instructors dead. It baffled Jake, as it did the other marines who heard of the shootings, that anyone would be foolish enough to give an Afghan, trainee or not, a full clip of ammunition. Thirty rounds was just so stupid. Anyone in the 1/5 would have handed out one or two rounds at most. That way if they turned on you they'd only be able to kill one or two before they'd run out of bullets. What had happened at that rifle range was Alice in Wonderland stuff. Those guys who had been killed hadn't even noticed that they had fallen down the rabbit hole.

The week Jake was promoted to corporal, he sent home a package of pictures that had been taken during his promotion while his unit was taking a rest and refit back at Camp Leatherneck. When his mother opened the envelope, the gritty dirt and dust of Afghanistan fell through her fingers onto the kitchen table. She stared at the small mound of grayish sand and started to cry.

17.

THAT DEADLY SENSE OF PRIVILEGE

Americans notice foreign policy only in the depths of a disaster
too colossal to ignore ... [there is] an evisceration of civic culture
that results when a small praetorian guard shoulders the burden of
waging perpetual war; while the majority of citizens purport to revere
its members even as they ignore or profit from their service ...

—Andrew J. Baceviche, Vietnam Veteran,
Professor Internal Relations, Boston College

Edward Gibbon said much the same thing in his *Decline and Fall of the Roman Empire.* Gibbon makes it clear that Rome succumbed to the barbarians due to a gradual decay of civic virtues among its citizens. He makes a special point of focusing on the outsourcing of the inherent duties to defend the empire as the beginning of the decline, ending with the fall of Rome as that abrogation of responsibility became institutionalized. What Gibbons documents was that within a period of sixty years not one general of the Roman Army and not one ground commander of any legion was from a family of wealth, privilege, or influence, even though these were the citizens who most benefitted from Roman power.

The military officers and, in growing numbers, the soldiers themselves were from the nations that Rome had subdued decades before. The Visigoths, the Gauls, the Germans, and the Huns gradually became the Romans who eventually did the fighting and eventually offered up Roman security out at the borders of the Roman Empire. Neither the nation detached from its army, nor the army detached from the nation, would survive.

As a people and as a nation, we have never endorsed the idea of a large freestanding army. It was Richard Nixon, angered with the growing resistance to our war in Vietnam, who supported and then promoted the idea of just such a volunteer army.

In a democracy, that old adage that "war is too important to be left to the generals" can become a two-edged sword. Politicians can be as foolish as any general, and faced with a population that is not involved or doesn't care that much about what is happening, can cause as much damage to a nation as any jingoistic military commander or field marshal.

Add to that mix of potential political or military hubris a volunteer army, removed from an unconcerned or uninformed electorate, pushed on by an imperial government or military establishment, and you have the ingredients for a national disaster; specifically, the implementing of narrow, self-serving decisions leading to ever-more widening unexpected and terrible consequences.

Indeed, it was to by-pass public scrutiny and possible opposition that the French Government, along with its military in 1831, formed the Foreign Legion so that they could send troops around the world, including Spain, Mexico, the African Colonies, Indochina, and Algeria, without having the French population become involved or even begin to think about their wars.

Our Revolutionary War has been our model. It has been the Citizen's Army we turn to in times of danger. Common sense has led us to believe that in times of real and actual danger, everyone must be involved, and a standing army simply would never offer up enough "boots on the ground" to win our battles, much less go on to win our wars.

Yet over these last decades we have become content to let such an army fight our battles, both out of sight and out of mind, under the foolish assumption that their will be no real individual or collective price to pay for it. We may not be Rome yet, but it is beginning to seem that way to the units that we keep deploying again and again, as well as their families and loved ones, while all the rest of us go shopping.

But it wasn't only two savvy Presidents, beat up by an anti-war movement energized by an unpopular draft, who clearly understood (from the most recently released White House tapes) that Vietnam was not going well and that we had to get out. A few of those generals who had served as company grade officers in World War II and Korea understood that a large part of that discontent and eventual antagonism to the war was that the country had grown disenchanted with the reasons we were fighting, coupled to a draft that was viewed as undemocratic and blatantly unfair.

The issue was never whether we should have a professional military. The country had decided that much in the 1850s with the establishment of West Point and Annapolis as training grounds for our officers. The question was who would pull the triggers and how the country would become committed to our future wars.

Among those generals trying to get it right was Creighton Abrams, who replaced General William Westmoreland as Commander of Military Forces Vietnam in late 1968. Abrams rethought the whole issue of public war and private commitment. Tough, crusty, and gruff, Abrams' concerns were quite different from both Johnson's and Nixon's, who wanted to get rid of a problem. Abrams simply wanted to get it right.

Abrams eventually came to view Vietnam as a war being fought by an army cut off from the population it served. What Abrams saw was that by 1969 the majority of combat units in Vietnam were made up mostly of minorities. He understood the inequality in all this and realized that this kind of smoldering demographic, barely working in a country at peace, could not work in a country involved in a deadly war that was going badly.

He became convinced that it was the separation of those who serve from those being served that had opened up the country to divisiveness, and the military to a conflict that had not been well thought out and, without public support, was ultimately doomed to failure. Abrams understood that the Vietnam draft had skewed conscription to the poor and disenfranchised, and away from those in positions of power, prestige, wealth, and privilege. He was aware of the long history of inequities in conscription, going back to the Civil War and Congress's 1863 legislation that allowed draftees to hire substitutes, paying a $300 fee to the government in order to avoid the whole conscription process. There was nothing so egregious or as flagrant as a $300 exception going on during the Vietnam War, but by the time Abrams took command of our troops there were no end to those same kinds of exemptions. There were undergraduate deferments and graduate school deferments. There were deferments for enlistment in the National Guard and Reserve units. There were medical deferments if you were connected enough to have a medical specialist document that you did have a certain degree of scoliosis or flat feet, whether you did indeed have asthma as a child rather than a chronic cough, or were so severely nearsighted that it was barely correctable by eyeglasses.

The three most famous cases of deferment during the Vietnam War years were those of two future presidents and a vice-president. George W. Bush spent his time during the war within the continental United States as a member of the Texas Air National Guard and Bill Clinton spent the war years with his own educational deferments at Georgetown and then at Oxford under the auspices of a Rhodes scholarship. Vice President Dick Cheney received five deferments during the Vietnam years, famously remarking that he had "other, more important things to do" at the time.

Abrams saw all this privilege as operationally hopeless and both politically dangerous and philosophically unsound. In response to this "privilege gap" and to make sure that it never happened again, Abrams' idea was for the country to maintain a small but competent volunteer army that would act as a powerful rapid deployment force to handle any fairly large-scale emergency. The plan was that for any prolonged conflict you could throw in the National Guard and Reserve units, giving America an immediate, quick, and abiding interest in any administration's continued pursuit of enlarging the military conflict. The idea was simple enough—calling up the Guard was sure to ensure a vigorous and lively national debate that would either end the conflict or legitimize and democratize the military effort by leading to the next obvious step, the establishment of a draft in order to continue the war.

Conceptually Abrams' plan was simple enough and there were many in the military, battered by the multiple failures of Vietnam, who went along with the idea. For anything more than a police action, the citizens of the country would become engaged through the activation and overseas deployment of their own state's National Guard and Reserve units, with a national discussion on reinstituting a draft sure to follow.

But it didn't turn out that way. By 9/11, we had a different kind of government, a different kind of army and apparently a different kind of country. There had been the success of Desert Storm I, and the Bush administration, with the Pentagon under Secretary of Defense Rumsfeld, was quite willing to let a small volunteer army, along with the addition of National Guard units to fill in the gaps, do the fighting. It would take Coleridge's "willing suspension of disbelief" for the country to look the other way when the caskets and wounded started to come home, and when more and more of those same units started being redeployed back into the war zones again and again. All the while believing that people who had been at each other's throats for centuries would suddenly embrace American-style democracy and welcome American troops as liberators. But it is the blindness or indifference of letting so few try to do so much while the rest of us went shopping that is the real tragedy.

Yet, even after a decade of fighting, with the volunteer army stretched to the limit and more and more reserve forces being deployed multiple times, no one is complaining, or even talking, of sharing the burden by instituting or considering a draft.

In 2006, Donald Rumsfeld, was asked by a relative of a deployed National Guard member why there were so many multiple deployments of Guard units, and why the National Guard troops were on operational duty, including foot patrols and setting up road blocks in the most dangerous districts and regions of Iraq. Unrepentant, unremorseful, and definitely annoyed, Rumsfeld answered dismissively, "The National Guard members knew what they were signing up for."

Well, not quite. Those Minnesota National Guard troops that I knew, many in their late thirties and early forties, some even in their fifties, had signed up for crowd control at celebrations, snow removal during blizzards, saving their neighbors during floods, and two weeks each summer at Camp Ripley swapping new stories with old friends. They had not signed up to kick in doors in the roughest neighborhoods in the world or drive down roads waiting to be blown up. Some 38 percent of all our troops in Iraq and Afghanistan have been and still are National Guard and Reservists. General Abrams would be surprised, maybe even astonished, but certainly disappointed that ten years into a war, the burden is on the military and not a generally involved and committed civilian population.

Colonel Harry G. Summers, in his book *On Strategy*, an analysis of the Vietnam War, wrote about the failures of the military in Vietnam that ring as true and as applicable today as when he wrote these sentences about a military some forty years ago:

Throughout the 1960s the military were torn between the commitment to civilian supremacy inculcated through generations of service and their premonition of disaster, between trying to make a new system work and rebelling against it. They were demoralized by the order to procure weapons in which they did not believe and by the necessity of fighting a war whose purpose proved to be increasingly elusive. A new breed of military officer emerged: men who learned the new jargon, who could present the systems analysis arguments so much in vogue, more articulate than the older generations and more skilled in bureaucratic maneuvering. On some levels it eased civilian-military relationships; on a deeper level, it deprived the policy process of the simpler, cruder, but perhaps more relevant assessments which in the final analysis are needed when issues are reduced to a test of arms ...

General Abrams died in 1974, having been given half his wish. We do have a small but powerful volunteer force, but the National Guard and Reserves are not supplementing the volunteer regular forces, they have been integrated into the force structure itself.

The air wing of the Minnesota Air National Guard flying C-130 has had multiple deployments to both Iraq and Afghanistan in order to fill in the gaps that an understaffed regular Air Force cannot supply. It is clear that our national amnesia has allowed a country of almost 300 million to allow fewer than 0.5 percent of the population, along with more than 300,000 women, to take on the whole burdens of what should be our fight in Iraq and Afghanistan.

For the last few decades economists have talked about the growing disparities between the rich and the poor in this country, the gentrification of American cities into the "haves" and "have-nots," along with the crumbling of the middle class and the growing gap between those with wealth and power and those without either. It is just this issue of class that Josiah Bunting III, a Vietnam veteran, novelist, and current president of the Harry Frank Guggenheim Foundation, addressed in his article "Class Warfare" published in *The American Scholar*. Bunting laments and warns about the loss of any sense of national duty and national service that has been swept aside by privilege and indifference. Bunting is unabashedly direct in his criticism of the nation's elite:

The business of war has become increasingly remote from a particular segment (the wealthy and the privileged) of the American people.

Bunting takes the issue of class further up the social ladder than most have been willing to go:

The war in Iraq (and Afghanistan) ... like Korea and Vietnam... has splintered away from the conscious concern of most of those in whose behalf it is said to be prosecuted.

He points out that those killed and wounded are no longer the children of those who lead this country, or, as Bunting writes:

Those who control its resources and institutions, dictate its tastes and opinions, and are blessed most abundantly with the country's bounty, or feed most lavishly upon its expensive entertainments and its treasures."

Bunting presents the record of one of this country's most prestigious but unnamed boarding schools. During World War I, 40 of its 400 students served in the military. During World War II, the number was 60. There were 10 during the Korean conflict, 5 for the ten years of the Vietnam War, and so far, none in Iraq or Afghanistan.

The 1956 Princeton graduating class sent a little less than half of its 900 graduates into the military, some as volunteers, some drafted within two years of graduation. In 2004, that same university sent 9 out of a class of 1,100. Today's Marines, patrolling the streets of Fallujah and the villages in Helmand Province, have the same attitudes, abilities, courage, and esprit de corps as the Marines of World War I and II, but today those prep school boys and Princeton graduates who had made up a significant part of those earlier units are missing. In 2007, the school sent almost 80 percent of its graduation class, not to Baghdad or Kandahar Province, but to Wall Street.

Bunting makes clear that the abandonment of a Citizen Army is the main cause for the national anesthesia concerning the wars in Afghanistan and Iraq. He points out that none of this is good for the country, the military, or our democracy. He ends his article with a statement written by George Washington at the end of his presidency:

It may be laid down as a primary position, and the basis of our system, that every Citizen who enjoys the protection of a free government, owes not only a proportion of his property, but even of his personal service, to the defense of it.

But Washington was not the only Commander-in-Chief who believed in Universal Service. The French General, Maurice De Saxe, who over a two-week period of illness in 1732 wrote down his views on war and a Citizen Army that was eventually published in his book, *Thoughts on the Art of War*. The book became to the military officers of the Eighteenth Century what Clausewitiz's *On War* was to become to the colonels and generals of the Nineteenth and Twentieth. Saxe's view on conscription, or the draft, in the chapter titled "On the Manner of Raising Troops" had clearly caught Washington's attention.

Would it not be better to establish by law that everyman, of whatever condition, was obliged to serve his prince and his country for five years? This law could not be objected to, because it is natural and because it is just that citizens exert themselves for the defense of the State. Choosing those between 20 and 30 years of age would result in no inconvenience—these are the years of license, where the young search for fortune, wander the country and are of no benefit to their parents. There would be no public desolation, as one would be sure that after the five years having passed, the young would be returned to their families. This method of raising troops would supply an inexhaustible fund of good recruits, not subject to desertion and by extension, cause it to be seen a duty and an honor to do one's part. But for success, it must be that no one of any condition be exempted, to be severe on this point, to be unmoving on its application to the rich and noble will ensure that none will complain. Those who have served their time will look with contempt on the Law's detractors and insensibly, it will become an honor to serve. The poor working man will be consoled by the example of the rich, the rich will dare not complain upon seeing the noble serve. Arms is an honorable profession. How many princes have borne arms. And how many officers have I seen serve in the ranks rather than live in indolence. It is only their weaknesses that make some view such a law as harsh.

Washington wrote his farewell speech 250 years ago, but the warning, if not the concern, is as real today as it was in 1793. Not to have some kind of personal involvement and even risk in issues of war and peace is to allow a kind of recklessness to enter those discussions that does not serve any real national purpose and is sure to end in both public confusion and personal tragedy.

These are the kinds of decisions that lead to what have been called "political wars," wars that are not fought for national security, but wars that are put into place for political or policy reasons rather than out of any real necessity. These political wars, usually trumpeted by policy hacks, offer only vague reasons for committing our armed forces, where any kind of winning is always hard to define and ultimate victory presented as some kind of distant far-off illusion. Because there is ultimately nothing important at risk, these are the wars that the politicians can offer up as wars that can be fought on the cheap. While real wars of necessity end in military victory or military failure, political wars usually end by everyone simply losing interest. Eventually, the tedium and casualties and the loss of treasure become too great to ignore, and the wars are simply abandoned and closed down while everyone pretends it wasn't that important. Or that none of it ever really mattered much anyway.

All of this simply walking away with nothing in hand makes the sacrifice of our troops and their families even harder to understand and much harder to accept.

It may be that in war or peace, the best way to focus the mind is to expose everyone's brain to real dangers. In the final analysis that may be the only way to make sure that wishful thinking is not replacing reality.

What is sure is that if there were a draft, all of America would know what John Witmer, author of *Sisters in Arms: A Father Remembers,* didn't know, and unfortunately, had to learn through a very steep and very tragic learning curve.

Mr. Witmer had no idea of the real dangers his daughters would face when they joined his state's National Guard. Like so many other Americans, he had no idea that hundreds of thousands of U.S. women had been deployed to Iraq and Afghanistan beginning in 2001. Like so many Americans, Witmer understood little about the military, less about our wars, and even less about who was doing the actual fighting. Witmer was certain that he, his wife, and their three daughters had nothing to fear when the girls joined the Guard. He assumed that the daughters, even when deployed to Iraq and Afghanistan, would not be put at risk. He was sure that as women, particularly women in the National Guard, they would be assigned to clerical work, doing typing and filing or to process, in and out, different pieces of equipment. It proved to be a fateful and fatal misunderstanding, one that he and his wife would have to live with forever. It never occurred to the Witmers that the girls were not clerk-typists sitting in an office but combat soldiers going out on combat raids and convoy protection missions.

One of John's daughters, the youngest, was manning a 50-caliber machine gun in the turret of an armored personnel carrier when she was hit by a sniper's round. The autopsy report that Mr. Witmer obtained some eleven months after her death stated that the bullet had entered her chest, passing directly through her heart, killing her instantly. What surprised him as he researched the facts surrounding his daughter's death was that the three other armored vehicles in the convoy all had women in the turrets manning the machine guns. Every automatic weapon in the three armored vehicles protecting the trucks in the convoy were manned by female soldiers. The inconvenient truth about Iraq and Afghanistan is that, without a draft, we have an army that cannot survive, much less fight, without women on the battlefield.

Women currently make up 20 percent of the 1.9 million troops that have been deployed into Iraq and Afghanistan and that percentage increases every month. That is our army now. And these are the soldiers our political leaders, and the country, have put in harm's way. But, as Bunting points out, these warriors are not their own daughters any more then they are their own sons.

If there were a draft, America, as well as the John Witmers, would have known that we have already deployed over a quarter of a million women to run the most dangerous roads in the world. They would know that more women have been killed and wounded in Iraq, and now in Afghanistan, then in all our other wars combined.

It would be known too, that those women who become amputees by losing an upper extremity are forced to choose hooks because most women in the military are less then 120 pounds and cannot carry the twenty-pound weight of the newest servo-magnetically-operated upper extremity prosthetic mechanical arms.

If there were a draft, Americans would know about women like Dawn Halfaker, a West Point graduate, who was severely wounded when an RPG came through the windshield of her Humvee, taking off the right arm of the platoon leader in the front seat and then continuing on through the vehicle, taking off her right arm at the shoulder. If that RPG had exploded, Dawn and everyone else in that Humvee would have been killed. Dawn spent a year at Walter Reed and today manages to deal with the ongoing phantom pain of her absent arm by exercising twice a day, using her own endogenous endorphin release to replace those doses of Percocet and Vicoden that had left her so groggy and at times so incoherent that she couldn't function. Years after her injury, she has basically made it on her own with the grit, determination, and toughness of a West Point graduate and a born athlete, along with the help of a few good friends.

If there were a draft, the country would surely know about Leigh Ann Hester, she would be a national hero. Sergeant Hester is the only woman to receive the Silver Star for valor since the Second World War. Sgt. Hester, at the age of twenty-three, and a handful of other Kentucky National Guardsmen fought off thirty insurgents armed with assault rifles, machine guns, and rocket-propelled grenades after the insurgents had attacked a supply column they were guarding. Hester, with one other Guardsman, killed twenty-seven of the insurgents, saving the column from destruction.

Sgt. Hester was a member of the 617 Military Police Company of the Kentucky National Guard. Before the Kentucky National Guard had been sent to Iraq, the unit's most dangerous duty had been crowd control at the Kentucky Derby.

It is not only that the last Administration never allowed photographs of caskets coming home, and ordered the planes flying the wounded into Andrews Air Force Base in Maryland to land only at night, or that the President never went to funerals of military personnel, or that the number of medals handed out for bravery are decidedly fewer in these wars than in any of our other wars. It is as if giving out medals for bravery might indicate that these wars are as ferocious and deadly as any of our other wars.

And that the real dangers of those we put in harm's way are decidedly greater than politically acknowledged or militarily reported. And all the sleight-of-hand appears to be going on as our newest President calls the escalating war in Afghanistan a War of Necessity. Well, if it is a necessity then we should all be involved and all begin to pay.

A surgeon stationed at the 24th Surgical Hospital in Balad in 2005 made a clearer statement about our latest War of Necessity:

There is no one with a lawn service who knows anyone in Iraq or Afghanistan.

18.

ALL THE CARRIES AND PRISCILLAS

Suddenly, a loud crash jolted them from their tranquil positions. A rocket-propelled grenade had just smashed the window and wall where the male marines were sleeping. Marine Lance Corporals Carrie Blais and Priscilla Kispetik dropped to the floor. "You okay?" they yelled to each other. Before they could grab their flak vests, Kevlars, and rifles, they heard the whistle of another incoming RPG and crash.

—*Band of Sisters: American Women at War in Iraq*,
Stackpole Books, 2007

Ask any ground commander in Iraq or Afghanistan and they will tell you, even as they remain professionally and publically silent, that our military could not function without its female soldiers and marines and not simply in support roles, but in actual combat. It is a fact that in wars with no front lines and even fewer secure areas, the differences between support and actual combat is at best illusionary and at worse uncompromisingly deadly. As a female soldier commented during the run up from Nasiriyah to Baghdad at the very beginning of Desert Storm II, " A missile doesn't target a specific gender."

Yet somehow as a nation and as individuals we seem not to understand the wars we are fighting and whom we are sending to make the fight. The idea that the Dawn Halfakers, Leigh Ann

Hesters, and the Witmer daughters are not the exception but the rule is part of the indifference of a country that is totally separated from those who decided to go to war and those we continue to send in ever-increasing numbers to get blown up on highways and mountain roads, go out nightly on dangerous raids, and daily have to fight their way out of ambushes.

The Marines have never experienced that confusion. They understand exactly the kind of fight we are in and who is doing the fighting and in their usual realistic uncompromising view of the world and of war understand what has to be done and more importantly how to do it. Of all the services, Army, Air Force, Navy, and Coast Guard, the Marines alone have refused to bend to feminist anger and, ignoring the accusations of political incorrectness, have done what they have always done and separated the sexes during basic training. A crusty old drill instructor gave the reason almost offhandedly in a conversation about women in the Marines. "The sexes differ in the need for their own types of endurance training as well as muscle building. The one-size-fits-all during basic training doesn't work any more. Hell, the V.C. and North Vietnamese troops probably weighed the same as our women do now and they beat us. It ain't the size that matters, it's the training. Besides, we know that sexual harassment is a problem and that there are long hours out on deployments in war zones or at permanent duty stations around the world right after basic. What we want is for one of our female marines to be able to say 'stop it or I'll kill you' and to have whoever is harassing her realize not only that she means it but that she can do it."

The sergeant was right on both counts. But what he also understood, though he might not have been able to put it into such clear-cut and definitive comments, was that this isn't World War II and the Norman Rockwell world of his past and ours has vanished for good, but his job remains what it has always been, to make sure his recruits, male or female, stay alive and are kept fighting. And in a way, his efforts have paid off.

The major cause of PTSD among female personnel in the Marines used to be sexual harassment. Today it is the same as male marines, namely, combat. This fact alone can be considered a success for women in the military, an equality based not on gender but on equal dangers and shared risks. While no one seemed to be looking, our armed forces have truly become equal opportunity organizations.

The refusal to believe or accept the fact that we routinely, and in ever-increasing numbers, send more and more of our women into harm's way, is as much a fantasy today as was the search for Weapons of Mass Destruction. We apparently have two parallel universes running side by side, one on the ground in Iraq and Afghanistan, and the other within the media and the rest of the country. And it is the issue of women in combat that may be the most compelling of the connections between the two and potentially the most contentious. It certainly will be the most illustrative of what has gone so wrong, and in the end, will probably end up saying more about us as a country than about policy, military strategy, and even day-to-day tactics.

It does take that poetic but real suspension of disbelief to walk down the street after ten years of wars that have sent over 300,000 women to fight in Iraq and now in ever increasing numbers to Afghanistan and see a young woman on a street corner missing an arm or walking on a prosthetic leg and automatically assume that it was because of a motorcycle accident. Perhaps America can be forgiven for not caring, but not knowing is a whole different matter.

In truth, the country, along with the military, has had a long history of ignoring or devaluing servicewomen. Until recently, women veterans have remained unrecognized while being treated as second-class citizens, even though many took on the risks and paid the price for being in combat.

It is not that women have not been acknowledged as warriors. There are archaeological findings from Fifth Century B.C, burial mounds in Southern Russia that Sarmatian and Scythian women did participate in wars. Up to 25 percent of military burials contain skeletons of armed Sarmatian women buried with their swords, lances, and bows. Certainly when the Sarmatian and Scythian men were away hunting or fighting, these nomadic women would have had to be able to defend themselves, their children, their animals, and their pasture grounds, not only competently but successfully.

It may well be that the Amazonian legend in Greek mythology was inspired by these real warrior women. But a race of Amazons cutting off their right breast to be better able to use a bow and killing all men except for procreation does not exist within the range of normal human experiences. Nevertheless, there remain enough archaeological signs throughout Central Russia and Asia Minor of female warriors dressed as men to authenticate the written accounts of the Greek historian Herodotus. But we don't have to go back to the Greeks.

Armed women have served as loyal bodyguards throughout the history of India. In medieval Scandinavia, women who did not have the responsibility of caring for a family could take up arms and live as warriors. Joan of Arc drove the English out of France. Throughout the late Nineteenth Century, the kings of Siam had a personal battalion of 400 spear-wielding women. And in the Twentieth Century, the Soviet Union began to train and incorporate women into the light infantry and the tank corps. But we don't have to go back to medieval France, Siam, or the Russians.

More than 20,000 women served as nurses in the American Expeditionary Force of World War I. They were subject to court-marshal authority, although they had no rank or military status. How many were wounded during those days of long artillery barrages or became casualties by being in ambulances carrying the wounded along back roads is impossible to discover. There is simply no official information on the number of women killed. It was not considered to be in the country's best interest to remind Americans that their women were being killed.

Over 400,000 women served in the military during World War II. Though these women were recognized for their contributions, any acceptance of their ability to do difficult or dangerous military work was ignored. And again, deaths and injuries were never rigorously documented or even discussed. That kind of reporting was considered at best "unseemly" and at worst counter-productive to encouraging national enthusiasm for the ongoing war effort. There were some things that you simply didn't talk about.

We won the war in both Europe and the Pacific and immediately began to disarm by emptying out the dozens of battle-hardened divisions. In 1948, with the Cold War heating up, Congress, aware of how our military had deteriorated since 1945, reluctantly turned to an untapped source of personnel and passed the first law allowing women to serve in regular peacetime forces. Necessity is indeed the mother of invention, or more accurately, of reality. But there were restrictions written into the law stating that women could not be promoted beyond the rank of captain in the Army, Air Force, and Marine Corps, and above the rank of lieutenant in the Navy.

We had a decidedly divided Army at the time, with most generals coming from the more conservative and traditionally-minded Southern States and most enlisted men from the North. It was the time of integration in the military and so the Pentagon, not so sure about putting blacks in positions of authority, took the worst of both these Americas—a South where the people didn't care how close a black man got as long as he didn't get too high, and a North that didn't care how high a black man rose as long as he didn't get to close, and applied both views to women.

The Pentagon did indeed finally let women into the armed forces, but at the same time restricted how high they could get and where they could go. Women in the Navy were barred from being assigned to ships other than hospital ships and Navy Transports, as if those ships could not be torpedoed or bombed, and from all potential combat missions.

Korea provided more combat experiences for another 120,000 women, as anyone watching the TV show *MASH* would understand. 10,000 service women went on to serve in Vietnam, with one reported death from enemy fire, despite the fact that during the Tet Offensive, on any number of the military bases being overrun by the Viet Cong, nurses as well as clerk-typists, female motor pool personnel, and intelligence specialists had to pick up weapons to fight beside their fellow male draftees and officers. Years later, the nurses, at least, received their own memorial at the Wall in Washington.

What is clear is that the years following Vietnam were a bad time for the military. Those remaining in the Army and the Marines during those rebuilding years were more concerned about reviving a dispirited and broken military, while focusing on institutional resurrection, and had little or no interest in experimenting with social engineering. But the Army had no choice.

The draft was gone and recruiting was terrible. With an attitude of "any port in a storm," the military did what they had to do and increased the numbers of women within its ranks. The Army decided and quite correctly, if still a bit gingerly, to use women, with their better education levels, test scores, and discipline, to help it transition to an all-volunteer force. There was little doubt though, that at the time senior Pentagon leadership thought of this as a temporary measure, pending the resumption, when necessary, of a future draft to adequately fill its officer and enlisted ranks with men. But again, and presumably into the future, women were banned from combat, but combat could not be banned from these women.

Vietnam had shown that in any future conflict there would be no clear front lines and no truly secure areas. It had also shown the dangers of not having enough troops on the ground, not sealing borders, not having an exit strategy, and not adequately training women for combat. But all these messages were to be lost on an Administration as well as a Pentagon some thirty years later.

Today those dangers are replayed daily in both Iraq and Afghanistan. This is a first hand account of what happens when you pretend not to be in combat when you are:

After searching the desert for a while, she found a burlap bag. Dig it up, someone said. She started digging and pulling until she couldn't pull any more. It was stuck. Then she noticed the wire coming out of it. "Put it down! Put it down!" the grunts yelled as they took off running in the opposite direction. She did as she was told and scampered away. Later, an EOD technician blew it up. It caused quite an explosion. If she had pulled any harder, she and those around her would have been toast.

That still goes on in Afghanistan. Life and death based solely on what you know and what you have been taught. Not to be trained for combat in a combat zone is a prescription for disaster.

The first Gulf War in 1991 pointed out the craziness of the no-combat directives for women. The established Pentagon "Risk Rule" at the time was that women could not be deployed in combat units such as the infantry, armor or artillery, but could be deployed in support units.

More than 40,000 servicewomen went to war and one out of every five women were deployed in direct support of combat units, though the distinction of combat versus support had grown decidedly fuzzier each week during that campaign, and would become more fuzzy with each subsequent war and each new deployment.

In the early 1990s, the *U.S.S. Eisenhower*, a navy aircraft carrier, received its first sixty women officers and enlisted personnel. They were not to be involved in combat operations, but sink an aircraft carrier and everyone on board sinks with the ship. During those years the three service academies also had become sexually integrated, giving the services a whole new cadre of competent female officers, while then Secretary of Defense Les Aspin opened combat aviation for the first time to women. The volunteer army needed bodies and some of the best bodies, as well as the best minds, were obviously female. The Pentagon understood that much about the wars we were to fight, even if the politicians had not yet caught on. When Desert Storm II began, the whole debate of whether women should be barred from actual combat took off again.

But operationally there was no turning back. The volunteer army had made fighting a war impossible without putting women at significant risk and our decisions to fight the kinds of wars we were actually going to have to fight were clearly forcing us to do just that.

From 2003 to the present, you would not find women in front line infantry units or driving tanks, but changes in technology and the very nature of our new wars had irreversibly blurred the definition of "being in combat." A number of women, like Leigh Ann Hester, who were in military police or other support roles, found themselves in vicious fire-fights and under attack by rockets and mortar as well as taking hostile fire while flying choppers across the wide expanses of Iraq and through the mountain passes of Afghanistan.

Women currently make up over 20 percent of the 1.9 million soldiers and marines already deployed to Iraq and Afghanistan. Between 2001 and 2009 over 200,000 female soldiers, marines and another 80,000 women from the National Guard and Army Reserves had been sent to the two war zones, with those numbers increasing every month. The absolute numbers and the percentages of women we have put in combat is simply astonishing, as are the risks they face.

The numbers of servicewomen killed is now approaching 700, as compared to one death in Vietnam, while the numbers of overall casualties—shattered limbs, penetrating head wounds, ruptured spleens and shattered kidneys, tension pneumothorax, traumatic brain injuries, burns, and PTSD—is passing levels of over 30 percent of all women deployed.

In World War II less than 0.2 percent of women in the armed forces were killed or wounded. In Iraq and now in Afghanistan, with the absolute number of troops deployed considerably less than the 13 million troops sent overseas in World War II, that number has reached 2 percent and is climbing towards 3 percent. The absolute numbers of women killed or wounded in Iraq and Afghanistan compared to the absolute numbers in World War II is more than staggering. When I ask audiences how many women do they think have been deployed to Iraq and Afghanistan since 2001, without even mentioning the fact that most are in combat, I get numbers of 500, 2,000, and the occasional 5,000. Nobody knows, because nobody has been told. The women know the risks, yet they continue to enlist.

Despite the obvious danger, the reason women join the military does not significantly differ from the reasons men enlist. But they do have more practical reasons for joining up. Title Nine, with the new acceptance and unembarrassed appreciation of the athleticism of young women, has something to do with it. These women can be recent high school or college graduates. They may need money for school. They may be seeking a career, want to do something fulfilling, or simply are looking for a challenge. Some want to follow in their father's footsteps, while many want to serve their country. Others want the excitement, and some just want a steady job with the world as the background. Those in the National Guard are for the most part single mothers who chose the Guard for the extra money and to do things for their neighbors, like flood control and helping out during winter blizzards. But the majority, Regular Army, Marines, or Air Force, are, in one way or another, using the military as much as a way up as a way out. But being a single mother in any of the services fighting in Iraq or Afghanistan brings a different kind of price to these wars.

New kinds of battles, new kinds of weapons, new kinds of strategies, and new kinds of tactics always bring new kinds of casualties. And our newest wars are no exception. In this war it is orphans, not their orphans, but ours. What is not in the records are how many orphans this war has left in its wake when those increasing numbers of single mothers are killed, or so severely damaged in mind or body they can no longer function as a parent when they finally do return home. It is as much a new legacy of these wars as the neurosurgical unit and the orthopedics wards. There are no numbers yet, but when this whole dark thing is over and the true data are finally compiled, those numbers will surely be in the thousands. A whole generation of children will be cared for by grandmothers, uncles, and aunts, all wondering how did all this happen.

Yet even today, the servicewomen sent to Iraq and Afghanistan, and in continually increasing numbers, still cannot drive tanks, but they can and do drive Humvees and trucks. And it is Humvees and trucks moving through the open deserts and along narrow mountain roads in long, exposed convoys that the Iraqis and Taliban target with mortars and small-arms fire, as well as ever more powerful IEDs that tear soldiers and marines apart. The Taliban, the Sunni Insurgents, and the Iranian-backed Shiites, along with their suicide bombers, do not make a distinction between servicemen and servicewomen, and perhaps neither should the military or our government.

We have chosen a volunteer army and without a draft that is the military we have and the one that we use. The distinction between female or male soldiers is a hold-over from some other age, like the nostalgia for the horse and buggy versus cars. It does not fit anymore but is itself dangerous. There are few soldiers currently on active duty in our war zones who do not fully accept women warriors within their ranks as long as they can pull their own weight. The angst about women in combat may be no more than the angst of those who simply cannot accept that biology is not destiny. But if we are going to choose to go to war and then send our soldiers and marines to make the fight, we should at least make sure that those we send, if not to win, at least know enough to stay alive and not get blown apart. Whether we like it or not, or admit it or not, our women are there, lots of our women, and we do have to train them as well as our men, and that training must deal with real combat and the ability to survive.

But nowhere is this lack of interest or concern more evident then in the VA system. Even with over 20 percent of those deployed to Iraq and Afghanistan being women and even with the vast majority being in combat, there are still no female clinics available to care for women with their different medical and surgical issues aside from their wounds and PTSD. Today across America, women walk into a VA hospital and are questioned by the guards and asked by intake workers, "Where is your husband?"

Still a good, if not necessary, beginning would be to give all the women in the military advanced infantry training. It makes no sense to put these women at risk and not give them the skills to make the fight and survive those risks. War does not give its participants time for on-the-job training. In Vietnam, new replacements were told to watch who'd been there a few months and do what they did. That was the training. If the new troops would do that, they had a chance to survive, if they didn't most would be dead before their first week was out.

Women have to be cross-trained in the use of all weapons, including the 50-caliber machine guns. They have to be taught how to use their radios to call for fire support, a basic and necessary military skill, but one that women are not taught or permitted to learn because it is a combat-related skill. Women should also be taught those basic skills on how to care for a gun-shot wound, as well as a leg or foot or arm that is blown off. The military has to teach these women how to fight, how to call in artillery and gunships, how to use all the weapons, and stop pretending that actual combat for them is not combat at all. Indeed, it would seem that everyone who is being shot at in either Iraq or Afghanistan understands that much about the reality of bringing democracy to the undemocratic.

But these are still women. That is always there. Erin Solaro, in her book, *Women in the Line of Fire,* mentions a female sergeant who, after a particularly vicious fire-fight, looks around at the marines policing up their gear and says with real affection "The marines are like little kids who need Ritalin." She paused, and flashing a small but satisfied maternal smile, clarified her comment, "The young ones anyway," she added, " those on their first combat tour …"

19.

BULLETS OF GRIEF / A PRESCRIPTION FOR PREVENTION

"We need a bigger bullet." What the young marine, just returned from Afghanistan, meant was a heavier bullet with more velocity, a longer range, and better terminal ballistics. More than one military surgeon had heard something like that during their own deployments, a few had heard it within weeks of the Iraq invasion in 2003.

The concern is no small thing. In our new kind of wars, the size of the bullet matters. During the battle for Telafar in 2005, General H.R. McMaster, then Regimental Commander of the 3rd Armored Cavalry, had issued M-14s, the successor to the Second World War's M-1 Garand rifle, to some squad members in each platoon.

The M-14 fires a much larger and heavier .308-caliber round that can reach out to ranges simply unreachable by the 22-caliber round fired from the standard-issue military M-4. In addition, a full .308-caliber round is able to penetrate cover that would deflect the M-4's smaller and lighter bullets. Anyone reading the After Battle Report would have guessed that, given the opportunity, the commander of the 3rd Armored Cavalry would have issued M-14s to all his troopers.

At the beginning of the war in Iraq, the Marines made the fight at Fallujah using the M-4. They would often hit insurgents with the smaller bullet but could not kill them or were unable to drop them. The insurgents kept attacking, at times bringing the fire-fights down to meters, and in a few places actually breaking through the Marine's forward positions. As one corporal put it, "They had to be hyped up on something. We'd hit them and they'd just keep coming."

This was something that hadn't happened to American Marines since they fought in the Philippines during the native uprisings in the late 1890s. At the start of the insurrection against American rule, the 38-caliber revolver, the standard-issue side arm for the Marines, was found to be unsuitable for the rigors of jungle warfare due to its unsatisfactory stopping power.

The weapon was upgraded to an automatic handgun firing a 45-caliber round. The heavier bullet was more effective against charging tribesmen who had high battlefield morale and used amphetamine-like drugs to inhibit sensations of pain. Yet, the message that bigger is better had gotten lost or was ignored as our armies moved into 1950s, 60s, and 70s.

Indeed, heavy-caliber rifle rounds had been standard issue since before the First World War. During the trench warfare of World War I, with most opposing forces well over 300 yards apart, if a soldier stood up or lifted his head out of the trench for a few seconds, he would be dead. Sergeant York, using a bolt-action M1903 Springfield rifle, firing a large caliber 30-06 round from over a third of a mile, single-handedly picked off a column of German soldiers one at a time, using a technique he had learned as a small boy hunting turkeys in the woods of Tennessee. He killed the Germans, as he had killed the birds, back to front to avoid alerting the German's at the front of the column.

It was a simple time, though I doubt that there was a physician in the U.S. Army units deployed to France who did not appreciate that degree of marksmanship.

Still, the ethical issues facing physicians in the military have not changed since medicine came to the battlefield. It is basically the result of that conflict between the Hippocratic Oath to heal the sick and relieve suffering, and General Patton's universal and timeless speech to troops that they were not there to die for their country but to make sure that the enemy died for theirs. What has added a modern edge to the reality of that tension is what a marine said to me some forty years ago at Zama and what they are still saying today, "We're the tip of the spear. Believe me, there isn't anyone out there trying to turn us into plowshares or pounding us into pruning hooks."

Whatever you may think, war is death and destruction and universally painful. Just as there are no atheists in a foxhole, there are no jingoists in a battalion aid station or a military triage area. What troubled physicians and surgeons in Vietnam who treated everyone brought into their hospital whether American, South Vietnamese, Viet Cong or NVA, is the same that troubles military physicians and surgeons in Iraq and Afghanistan today. With the escalations in deaths and casualties as troop numbers are increased, the same realization comes into play, if anyone is going to have to be killed or wounded, better it be them than us. It is a desperate Hobson's choice with no clear cut or acceptable default position.

How to hold both the Hippocratic Oath and the reality of war in the same breath, not to mention the same mind, is at best a difficult and perhaps impossible task. Ultimately, you have to pick a side or you just have to stay clear of the whole thing. That is the choice. Still, like any reasonable medical or therapeutic decision, the facts help.

Regarding the bullets, those facts and that history are as simple as they are clear. You either have the right bullet or you don't, and if you don't the whole ethical issue quickly morphs into something decidedly less slippery than ethics—responsibility. And that anyone can understand and hopefully appreciate. We simply need to give our troops a bigger bullet.

Whatever else might be said about World War I, it was a war where marksmanship, accuracy, the hitting power of large-caliber bullets, as well as the operational range of the rifle, mattered as it had in every war since the invention of firearms. At Gallipoli in 1916, the average life span of an Australian or New Zealand soldier moving about outside of the trenches was somewhere in the neighborhood of one to two minutes. That in itself, after six months, ended the campaign, with the Allied Forces simply giving up and going home. But things were changing. Technology was taking over, not only within civilian industry, but within militaries themselves.

The last years of the First World War saw the development of a number of fully-automatic weapons, including the 1919 Browning automatic rifle, the Thompson submachine gun, the German machine pistol, and the British Vickers machine gun. The industrial revolution had been in place for some sixty years when World War I began and so it was time for slaughter on an industrial scale.

These automatic weapons fired a shorter and slightly lighter bullet than the standard 30-caliber rifle round. The lighter bullets allowed these automatic weapons to fire a large number of rounds, without substantial recoil, over a very short period of time. The soldiers using these weapons, however, had to carry the increased numbers of cartridges needed to fire these weapons. The arguments then are the arguments used today to justify the use of the lighter, less kinetic, rounds in both Iraq and Afghanistan.

What is not arguable is that the "lighter" ammunition combined with the automatic fire did away with *aiming*, and the issue of marksmanship quickly morphed into a new military doctrine of "Spray and Pray." Enamored by the numbers of rounds that could be fired per minute, this new doctrine replaced individual expertise and personal battlefield skills with sheer volume. Like so much that has happened with industrialization, the machine replaced craftsmanship.

Still, that idea of not aiming was a potential problem which the military did understand, and dealt with by taking the full auto-setting off the upgraded M-16s and M-4 to allow for single shot or 3-round bursts. Yet, the development of the assault rifle by virtually every major military in the world was the modern battlefield answer to the balance between a rifle that, if aimed properly, was able to fire long distances and still drop whoever was hit, with the sustained rapid fire of the automatic weapon used at close quarters.

All the assault rifles used the smaller reduced 30-caliber cartridge, universally called the 5.56 round, that contained less powder than the original larger and heftier 30-caliber rifle cartridge. The German assault rifles developed for use on the Eastern Front at the close of the Second World War used a larger 30/08 or 7.92-mm round based on the full powder, older 30-caliber cartridge. Yet, only a few hundred thousand of these assault rifles were ever issued to German forces. Consequently, the only units of the German Army to successfully fight their way out of the encircling Red Armies throughout 1944 and early '45 were those units that had been issued the assault weapons firing these larger rounds. The German units firing assault rifles using the more powerful cartridges were able to kill more Russians, at a farther distance, than the Russians were able to kill Germans at those same distances, using automatic weapons with the lighter cartridges.

Despite all the technology, there are still times out on the battlefield—and more often than has been or is currently being admitted—when surviving the life and death struggles of modern warfare may mean no more than using a bullet a few hundred grams heavier, with greater terminal ballistics, than the bullet your enemy is using. That was a message that somehow has gotten lost. It made a difference in World War I and World War II and once again today can mean the difference between living and dying.

In the early 1940s, the U.S. military believed there was a need for a light carbine to be used by personnel not in direct combat, that offered more personal defense than the standard issue 1911 / 45-caliber Colt pistol developed in the Philippines during the native insurrection and used throughout World War I.

The carbine worked well for close-in defense and limited assaults against lightly fortified positions. In these limited encounters the carbine, firing little more than a slightly more powerful handgun cartridge, was definitely better than using a pistol. But in Korea, the carbine proved a deadly nightmare for U.S. troops.

The Chinese, attacking in winter across the frozen Yalu River at the Chosin Reservoir, wore padded winter uniforms. More than one marine was killed, who after putting a few rounds from a carbine into a Chinese soldier who did not drop, kept up the attack. Faced with these lighter rounds, the Chinese in their padded winter uniforms might just as well have been wearing Kevlar vests. There were instances during the Korean War of our troops simply throwing away their carbines and looking for an M-1 Garand or a Browning automatic rifle or even an M-14, in order to stay alive.

It would not have been unreasonable for the physicians in the MASH Units—and there was a script that had been in the works for the TV show *MASH*—to make the point to their more senior officers that if they didn't want their soldiers and marines killed and wounded they would have to dump the carbines and distribute weapons that would work. Preventive medicine is still a part of medicine in general and it is certainly a part of military medicine, whether issuing tablets to fight off malaria or adding iodine tablets to make contaminated water potable. Unfortunately, history was doomed to repeat itself.

In the middle 1950s, the U.S. Army established a program to develop weapon systems based on the combat statistics of World War II for what was called the "Battlefields of the Future." The data showed that the greatest number of kills from small arms had occurred at less than 300 yards, with the majority to be within 100 yards of enemy combatants. It was determined that the military should consider very light-weight, high-capacity weapons that would be effective at close ranges, especially less than 100 yards. Once again, it was explained that the use of lighter rounds would allow soldiers to carry more ammunition, while firing a less kinetic bullet would provide controllability to the weapons, even under full automatic fire.

U.S. military doctrine now called for being able to carry enough rounds so that a soldier could keep firing until he finally hit someone or something. Long standing factors such as aiming and distances were disregarded. The analysts were now in charge. "Spray and Pray" had become Pentagon policy, but with even more spraying and more praying, at the time, no suitable cartridge was available for that proposed new small-caliber assault rifle.

But Eugene Stoner, while working at the Armlite Corporation on just such a weapon, looked at the then available 22-caliber cartridges and based on the slightly heavier Remington Magnum 22-caliber round, developed the lightweight but more powerful, NATO-designated 5.56-mm rifle cartridge for his new rapid fire AR 15 assault rifle. Virtually overnight a star was born. The production of the AR 15 Stoner rifle was leased to the Colt Company and produced by the millions as the Military M-16.

Rushed into production in the middle 1960s for the Vietnam War, the physics of initial velocity and end-point ballistics soon caught up with the new weapon and the new round. Even though the 5.56 cartridge was lightweight, had low recoil, and met the absolute military specifications of being able to penetrate a steel helmet at 300 yards, the round did not have the reach of the other older and heavier military cartridges. Additionally, there was the problem of knockdown power. The 5.56, which despite its increasing powder load, was still a 22-caliber round and lacked the energy to reliably knock down a determined or crazed attacker past 100 yards.

The Soviet Bloc countries, as well as their allies and surrogates, had also drifted to fully automatic weapons, but used a much heavier 30-caliber round. The famous AK 47 was the product of this type of assault rifle.

But across the world, updated versions of the old-fashioned bolt-action World War I rifles were used by snipers, commandoes, and Special Forces, as well as nuclear weapon guards. These are considered critical military specialties where the target has to be killed. These are weapons to be used in situations where there was not the luxury of a second chance. That should have told our military something about the realities of combat. More times then anyone is willing to admit, there is never that luxury of a second chance.

Nowhere are the limitations and dangers of the Stoner 5.56 round more clearly or more dramatically described than in Kent

Anderson's book on the Special Forces, *Sympathy For The Devil,* where two special forces officers getting drunk at a bar in Da Nang during the beginning of the Vietnam War discuss the differences between their M-16 cartridge and the AK rounds they are up against.

Hanson was standing next to the bar. "You know," he said, holding a bullet in each hand between thumb and forefinger, "you can get an idea of a country's national character by the bullets their armies use."

"Oh, yeah," Quinn said, turning on the bar stool to look at Hanson. "I guess you're going to tell me about it."

"Now you see," Hanson said, "here's the standard American small-arms round," and held up the bright bullet toward Quinn. "It's slim, lightweight, and fast, but unstable. Look at it," he said, shaking the pencil-thin round. "It's the bullet equivalent of a fashion model—sexy-looking, thin, glittering. But if it gets dirty or damp or overheated, it's liable to jam on you. Temperamental, a prima donna.

"Now here's the Russian bullet," he said, holding out the dull AK-47 round. "Short, thick around the middle. The peasant woman of bullets. Sturdy and slow, not easily deflected by brush, dependable at long range. You can stick it in the mud, put it in the gun, and still shoot it."

"We're shooting our fashion models at them and they're firing back with peasant women," he said, holding out the bullets, grinning.

A battalion surgeon with the 9th Division in the Delta or a medic up in the Central Highlands could not have said it better. Erin Solaro, in a recent interview about women in combat, gave a clearer view while adding a bit of feminine testosterone to the controversy:

The cartridges used in the M-16 in Vietnam and the same 5.56 round used in the M-4s in Iraq and Afghanistan are a bunch of shit.

A soldier having spent two tours in Iraq and recently one in Afghanistan said much the same thing:

We're using varmint rifles and they're using real guns. We try to get assigned to the .50 Cals that way we can kill 'em and don't have to worry about having to hit them with three rounds before they drop. Believe me, we complained but no one listened.

Yet, even while Stoner was willing to give away distance based on the Army's own data on most kills being at less than 300 yards with the majority of those under 100 yards, he clearly understood the physics of bringing a smaller bullet to what were surely to be deadly gunfights. He understood that the low kinetic energy of his 22-caliber round would become a real survival issue once they were used in actual combat.

In the military, a soldier or marine should be able to drop anyone he or she hits. There is no place in a battle for a fair fight. In any combat situation, a soldier doesn't want to give the enemy a break and he certainly doesn't want anyone he shoots to keep moving—much less be able to shoot back.

So Stoner did the obvious. A physicist at heart, he started to fiddle. He increased the hitting power of his new bullet by actually decreasing the rifling of the M-16 barrel so that the bullet was spinning at a slower rate when it left the barrel of the gun, making the bullet barely stable in flight almost from the moment that it left the barrel. Most middle or long-distance weapons have a ten or eight twist to length rifling of the barrel in order to keep the bullet spinning fast enough to maintain a stable trajectory. That twist to length rifling allows the round to reach out accurately and predictably to considerable distances without fluttering off course, being deflected by windage, or losing significant terminal energy as it hits the target.

The degree of spin acts like a gyroscope, keeping the bullet on line and stable in flight. Stoner's reducing of the twists in the barrel of the M-16 allowed the bullets to quickly tumble and a tumbling bullet, even with losing energy, can still cause terrible wounds that become the classic "small hole in/big hole out" wounds.

But tumbling bullets are also easily deflected. It is the reason that soldiers in 'Nam out on patrol were relieved to have someone on point with a sawed off shotgun or a cut down M-60 machine gun that could fire rounds through tangled jungle growth and kill anyone off the trial waiting in ambush.

Stoner had also expected that distance would not be a big problem in the jungles of Southeast Asia. And for the most part he was right. But those shortcomings of the M-16 became obvious during the First Iraq War. The war was won quickly but, out in the open reaches of desert and long sight lines of central Iraq, the majority of engagements were at distances not experienced since the trench warfare of World War I.

The M-16 needed greater reach. The military tightened the twists within the barrel and redesigned the bullet up from 55 to a weight of 62 grains. While making the cartridge more powerful, the military added a steel tip to the round, making the bullet lighter in the front and forcing the bullet to be intrinsically unstable so that it would wobble as it was spinning faster and reaching out to longer distances.

But despite the readjustment, the give and take of physics goes to work. The now heavier bullet had a slower exit velocity, losing significant terminal energy the longer out it reached. The now rapidly spinning bullet didn't always tumble as expected. In short, many of the hits from the newly designed M-16 round, while reaching further out, resulted in a small hole in, as well as a small hole out, leading to little, if any, internal damage other than along the track of the bullet. If the round did not hit a vital organ, break a bone, or cut a major artery, the person hit simply kept moving.

The government and the Pentagon never acknowledged the problem or the danger to our troops. In the early 1990s, the standard M-16 was reincarnated into the M-4 weapon system. The M-4 is similar to an earlier compact model M-16 and still fires the 5.56 round. But it is a more convenient weapon than the full-sized M-16 to carry in cramped areas like tanks, trucks,

Humvees, and Armored Personnel Carriers, while its smaller size makes it easier to use in the buildings, narrow streets, and alley-ways of urban centers. But both the compact M-16 and the M-4 have a decidedly shorter barrel than the full sized M-16 and that shorter barrel means less initial exit velocity, and even less kinetic energy for the 2.23 cartridge.

Once again, physics plays its own nasty game. The shorter barrel has the consequence of slowing the exit speed of the bullet. The speed of a bullet increases as the bullet is pushed forward down the barrel by the expanding gases of the cartridge. Shorten a barrel for any reason and the amount of time the bullet is exposed to the expanding gases decreases, and the slower the bullet is moving as it exits the rifle, the lower the terminal velocity.

Surprisingly, this sacrifice in exit velocity and the decrease in terminal ballistics, in exchange for the ease of handling of a weapon, are considered to be a worthwhile compromise. There is no doubt that the M-4 is an adequate weapon for troops under close conditions. But for shooting at enemy forces at middle and long distances or trying to fire at insurgents behind rocks and stone walls, most troops would rather have a 30-caliber round and a rifle with a longer barrel.

Those who have made the fight in Iraq and Afghanistan understand that we have come full circle and that, in order to win these wars, at least down at the platoon and company-sized firefights, we have to go back to World War I and have a weapon in our arsenal that can be aimed and is both accurate and deadly out at long distances.

The refusal to do this is undoubtedly due to sheer exhaustion. We are still reeling from how we got into all of this and how unprepared we were for what actually happened. The result is an Army and Marine Corps that is stretched too thin.

Secretary of Defense Robert Gates, who will retire this year, and so can speak openly, recently expressed both the country's and the military's confusion, "This war will always be clouded by how it began." And so these wars remain clouded not only as to how they should end but how they should be fought.

Bob Woodward's newest book, *Obama's War*, describes Vice President Biden's trip to Iraq and Afghanistan right after the 2008 presidential election. As Woodward describes the three-day trip, the Vice President, in his usual loquacious way, asked everyone he met, particularly the commanders in the field, how they thought things were going and how they thought things could be improved. He became distressed as he gradually realized that the commanders making the fight had no real idea why they were there, what the exit strategy was, and more importantly, what victory or even defeat would actually mean. Woodward makes clear that Biden is eighteen years older than the President and adds to the description of the trip that the majority of commanders viewed the Karzai government as corrupt and that Biden, remembering Vietnam, could not help but think that this was Vietnam all over again.

The military's effort in all this has been directed to trying to get its mission right amid the confusion of changing goals such as counter-insurgency, counter-terrorism, nation-building, democracy or federalism, staying as long as necessary, or leaving by a certain date.

All this shifting about has made changing a major weapon system given to our 4.5 million regular duty military, national guard, and reserve personnel an enormous task. It could only be considered a further kind of tinkering to a military trying not to look foolish and actually trying to survive. The armament industry, with its lobbyists and consulting retired generals and colonels, are all too willing to go before Congress to testify that our weapons are the best in the world, while explaining that they are effective if used correctly and within approved guidelines. And those on active duty who are running the roads and working in the Afghan mountains do not have the time, the energy, or the clout to make that kind of fight to make things right.

But for those in the business of saving lives and trying to make people whole again it is not only necessary, but an absolute requirement, to tinker down at the very tip of the spear.

Afghanistan may not yet be Vietnam, but neither is the new Taliban the old Taliban. Those now fighting in Afghanistan are no longer disorganized insurgents trying their luck at playing soldier. The most recent Taliban attacks are coordinated and militarily sophisticated. Our own military responses have to be more immediate, more formidable and more deadly. Today there is even more of a value in engaging the enemy at a distance as well as being able to kill them at close quarters. And for that—we need a larger bullet.

Upgrading our M-4s would mean little more than changing the barrels, as well as altering the receivers to accept a larger round. It would be expensive. But so are the orthopedic wards at Walter Reed, the Rehab Center at Brooks Army Hospital in Texas, and the Poly-trauma Units at the VA hospitals across the country.

But there is a more immediate and decidedly cheaper answer to the whole issue of a better weapon for the 50,000 troops we will be leaving behind in Iraq and the 150,000 troops in Afghanistan. The military will have to unwind its history of the last half dozen decades and ignore that "Spray and Pray'" approach to the use of individual weapons, and go back to having our troops look at what they want to shoot and then reach out and hit those who have been targeted.

William Langewiesche, international correspondent for *Vanity Fair*, in his article "The Distant Executioner," published in February 2010, tells the story of what is happening today in our military regarding its weapon systems and what must happen in the future. Langewiesche would hardly view his article as an essay on preventive medicine but that is precisely what it is. There is a great deal more Patton than Hippocrates in what today's military physicians are forced to deal with and have to face on a daily basis. But then again, Patton knew a great deal more about war than Hippocrates.

According to Langewiesche, there are fewer than 2,000 fully-trained snipers in the Army and National Guard, fewer than 800 in the Marines, and a few dozen in the Air Force and

Navy. Yet, when he interviewed those officers making the fight in Iraq and now in Afghanistan, it was clear that these specialists are considered to be valuable assets, but still too scarce to be assigned to regular front line units.

The solution Langewiesche presents is basically to train more front line troops to act as "snipers" and give them the sniper's favorite bolt-action Remington rifle using a large 30-caliber round, and then add those who become qualified to the inventory of every squad, or, at the very minimum, to every platoon in the military that is or will be sent to Iraq or Afghanistan. As the author points out, a new Military Occupational Specialty classification or MOS of "Marksman," to go along with the other military specialties from Radio Operator to Medic, would ignore the atmospherics that go with the current MOS of "Sniper."

What is implicit in the article is that the addition of a single marksman to every operational unit gives the necessary reach our troops need for both personal and unit security. The added implication to that important factor is that crucial dimension, absolutely critical to winning the hearts and minds of those in a war zone, of not shooting what shouldn't be shot and not killing who shouldn't be killed.

There is an irony in all of this. We have a high-technology army with ever-increasing, computerized, real-time battlefield situational awareness, unmanned drone flights that fire on-demand hell-fire missiles guided by an operational command center in Fort Bliss, Texas, cell phone intercepts, and high-resolution satellite imagery used to pin-point potential military targets. In the midst of all this, a single marksman using a high-power scope and firing a single heavy .308-caliber bullet from a bolt-action Remington 700 rifle may actually be both our newest, as well as our best, secret weapon.

We may have come full circle, though the physician's role in all of this hasn't changed over the decades, much less over the centuries. It is what it has always been, to save those who can be saved and try to fix those who can be fixed. But it has also been to bear witness. Medicine has never offered immortality, but it has offered relief from suffering, as well as an understanding of grief and loss. But at its best, medicine has offered prevention and concern for each individual patient. That too is part of the Hippocratic Oath.

It is not the least bit ironic, nor a stretch, but with prevention and individual concern in mind, the addition of marksmen to every unit in Iraq and Afghanistan, along with increasing the caliber of the bullets used by all the troops, may well be the best medicine for those we send to make our fights—other than never having sent them in the first place.

20.

"IS MY JUNK ALL TOGETHER?"

Everybody was taken aback by the frequency of these injuries: the double amputations,the injuries to the penis and testicles. Nothing like this has been seen before ... unbeliveable.

—Dr. John Holcomb, retired Army Colonel

Since the surge in Afghanistan of 30,000 new troops in 2010 along with the new emphasis on counterinsurgency—the winning of hearts and minds through foot patrols in order to get to know the villagers—rather than the counterterrorism strategy of simply killing the bad guys, the surgeons caring for our wounded are beginning to speak of a new kind of "signature wound". New tactics and new strategies always lead to new kinds of injuries.

These wounds have been seen before but never in such numbers that they can no longer be ignored or explained away as just bad luck. As one of the military trauma surgeons recently offered, "I've seen these types of injuries before. What I haven't seen is them coming in over and over and over again."

The new signature wound is a composite injury and usually the result of a soldier stepping on a buried land mine. It is two legs blown off at the knee or higher with severe damage to the genitals, colon, rectum, and bladder. Multiple limb amputations have always been a part of the fight in Iraq and Afghanistan, but these genital wounds resulting in the loss one or both testicles while requiring colostomies as well as bladder reconstructions all taken together in the same patients is something new. But put your troops on the ground as foot patrols walking into and around villages or across farm compounds and these are the wounds you get. In addition, a number of these patients require "hip disarticulations"—the removal of the entire thigh bone, which makes the use of a future prosthesis at best problematical if not actually impossible.

The surgeons at Landstuhl Regional Medical Center in Germany where virtually every severely wounded soldier and marine is sent on their way back to the States must have felt much like Ambroise Paré in the 16th Century when Paré was forced to deal with the shattering injuries from gunshot wounds.

The problem was the body armor. The armor clearly reduced fatalities and the triangular flap on the lower part of the armor protects the groin from projectiles coming from the front, but does not protect the legs nor the areas between the legs, specifically the genitals, the bladder, and rectum from any upward moving blasts or projectiles.

The army has been reluctant to acknowledge these new types of wounds through some fear of giving the enemy information and potential insights into making their IEDs and other weapons even more effective. But the troops know. With the numbers of wounded losing one or both testicles on the rise, those who have been deployed are telling those who are to be deployed to store some of their sperm at home before they leave the States for the mountains and plains of Afghanistan.

This is not a foolish concern. An intensive care nurse at Landstuhl explained the new reality. Those most severely injured arrive at Landstuhl unconscious or heavily sedated, usually regaining some consciousness within two to three days. "The first thing we let them know is they are in Germany. We tell them that they are hurt but okay." The first question the wounded then ask, even before they check for their arms and legs—"Is my junk all together?"

The soldiers and marines know at least one of the real outcomes of a counter-insurgency that relies on foot patrols in a landscape set up for war. There is currently nothing in the medical literature about the long-term care, the effectiveness of the different male hormone-replacement therapies, quality of life issues, or the psychological adjustments for injuries that cause the destruction of or damage to the male sexual organs. But someone is going to have to figure all this out and figure it out quickly because these kinds of wounds are not going away and will only increase in number the longer we stay in those mountains and valleys.

21.

CHRONICLES / REDUXING VIETNAM

This summer over 2,300 years ago, Alexander the Great, after conquering most of the known world, barely makes it out of Afghanistan into India through the Hindu Kush with less than a third of his army by marrying the daughter of the Northern Afghan Chieftain. When you look at a map of the conquests of Genghis Kahn in the Thirteenth Century—the lands conquered in blues and greens—everything from China, the Russian Steppes through the Middle East, and half of Europe is in color except a tiny white circular dot below the Himalayan mountains that represents today's Afghanistan.

In 1842, during the Second Anglo-Afghan War, all of the 20,000 British troops sent there in what Kipling called "The Great Game of Politics" were killed in the mountain passes above Kabul with only one officer, a physician, making it out of those mountains.

The Soviet Union invaded Afghanistan on Christmas Day, 1979 and left nine years later in February of 1989. The Russians had ended up with over 250,000 troops in Afghanistan with absolutely no rules of engagement. They could kill anyone and destroy any village they chose—and they did.

Over that nine-year period, a million Afghans were killed and another 3 million became refugees, and yet, like every other invading army, the Russians eventually had to leave. Afghanistan is a tough place to fight and even a tougher place to win. The landscape is set up for war.

In recently released transcripts of Politburo meetings in the winter of 1986, three years before the Soviet leaders pulled the Russian Army out of Afghanistan, Sergei Akhromeyev, commanding the Soviet Armed Forces, explained the problems his soldiers were facing fighting in the hills around Kabul, as well as in the Kandahar and Helmand Provinces now occupied and patrolled by U.S. troops.

"Our soldiers are not to blame," Marshall Akhromeyev made clear. "They've fought incredibly bravely in adverse conditions. There is no piece of land in Afghanistan that has not been occupied by one of our soldiers at some time or another. Nevertheless, much territory stays in the hands of the terrorists."

"We control the provincial centers, but we cannot maintain political control over the territory we seize. To occupy towns and villages temporarily has little value in such a vast land where the insurgents can just disappear into the hills. ... 99 percent of the battles and skirmishes that we fought in Afghanistan were won by our side. The problem is that the next morning there is the same situation, as if there had been no battle. The terrorists are again in the village where they were—or we thought they were—destroyed a day or so before."

Marshall Akhromeyev went on to request extra troops and equipment.

"Without them, without a lot more men, this war will continue for a very, very long time."

Before the invasion, the Chief of the Soviet Defense Staff, Marshal Nikolai Ogarkov, had raised doubts about the invasion. He had told Dmitri Ustinov—then defense minister —"that the experience of the British and Czarist armies in the Nineteenth Century should encourage caution."

A review of history should have cautioned anyone thinking of invading those mountains or those plains of Afghanistan. Why it didn't cause us to hesitate remains an abiding mystery. It may simply be Arthur Schlesinger's warning about those four most dangerous words in the English language, "This Time It's Different," again being ignored.

The Russians continued their war for three more years before they finally withdrew from Afghanistan and went home. In fact, before the withdrawal in 1989, there had been a military recommendation for a "surge," Soviet style.

The equivalent of the head of the Russian Joint Chiefs of Staff had suggested sending in the whole of the Russian Army. The transcripts reveal that Mikhail Gorbachev, who had become the Russian leader in March of 1985 and had privately begun calling Afghanistan "our bleeding wound," would have none of it. There was to be no surge. Gorbachev eventually opted to pull out the troops and go home. At the same time that Gorbachev was trying to decide how best to deal with his disastrous war, Anatoly Chernyayev, his chief foreign policy aide, was writing in his own personal diary that Afghanistan had become *"Our Vietnam. But worse."*

EPILOGUE

Today in Afghanistan, with IEDs becoming the Taliban's weapon of choice, those injuries that do not kill our Marines outright or cause traumatic brain injuries will inevitably lead to multiple amputations. Troopers on foot patrol often lose both legs and one arm from the blast. We all walk with our arms swinging, whether it is down the block in front of our homes or on patrol outside of a supposed Taliban village. In Afghanistan, the body usually shields one arm whether the blast is behind, to the side, or in front of the marine.

To deal with these injuries, the military has recently developed a new kind of tourniquet specific for Afghanistan called a CAT or "Combat Action Tourniquets." Two CATs are now being issued to every marine going to or already in Afghanistan. Each CAT has a black plastic cinch device around it that when pulled, tightens the tourniquet, cutting off the blood supply to the damaged or missing limb.

Today the marines in Afghanistan who go out on foot patrols go out with the tourniquets already loosely strapped high on their thighs so that the tourniquets can quickly be tightened immediately after a leg or a foot is blown off. No one ordered the marines to go out with tourniquets already in place. Abandoned in "The Grave Yard of Empires" they have simply decided on their own to give themselves the chance of at least going home alive.

*****

In May of 2010, the number of American dead in Afghanistan passed 1,000 after a suicide bomber in Kabul killed at least five United States service personnel. The ages of those killed clearly show that American troops are dying younger, often right out of boot camp. The apparent reason that the age of those killed in Afghanistan is dropping is that the pool of experienced combat troops is shrinking. Without a draft, the military has to send younger and less experienced soldiers and marines into the fight.

From 2002 to 2008, the average age of service members killed in action in Afghanistan was twenty-eight; in 2009, that age quickly dropped to twenty-six. This year, the 125 troops killed in combat had an average age below twenty-five. These are getting close to Vietnam ages. The other number that is similar to 'Nam is that the incidence of those killed to those wounded is going up as the number of IED attacks increase and the devices themselves become more powerful.

More of our troops are killed right then and there when the IED explodes, rather than being wounded. A bomb estimated at over 2,000 pounds recently killed seven American soldiers riding in a troop carrier. No one survived long enough to make it to a med-evac chopper, much less a hospital. That too is like 'Nam. Dead the moment you are hit.

ACKNOWLEDGMENTS

Thanks to Bob Aulicino for a cover that captured the book, Angela Werner for her tireless editorial efforts, Kendra Millis for the indexing that mentions everything worth mentioning, and my agent Claire Gerus who brought the manuscript to publisher Don Bracken, who saw a book he had to publish.

GLOSSARY

AK-47 – Communist 7.62-mm semi-automatic and fully automatic assault rifle

AK-50 – The newest version of the AK-47. Some have a permanently mounted "illegal" triangular bayonet, which leaves a sucking wound that will not close.

AOD – Administrative officer on duty

APC – Armored personnel carrier

AR – Army regulation

ARVN – Army Republic of Vietnam

Bandoliers – Belts of machine-gun ammunition

Boonies – The countryside

Bouncing Betty – A mine with two charges: one to propel the explosive charge upward and the other set to explode at about waist level.

Bravo – Army designation for infantry man

Burr Holes – Surgical holes drilled through the skull so that the brain and its surrounding vessels can be operated on.

CA – Combat assault. Term applied to taking troopers into a hot landing zone.

Chopper – Helicopter

Cobra – Heavily armed assault helicopter

CP – Command post

Dust Off – Medical evacuation mission by helicopter. The term refers to the great amount of dust thrown up by the rotors as the med-evacs come in to land.

Enucleation – Surgical removal of the eye

ENT – Ear, nose, and throat

Fire Base – An artillery battery set up to give fire support to surrounding units

FO – Forward observer

Grunt – Originally slang for a marine fighting in Vietnam, but later applied to any soldier fighting there.

H and E – High explosive

Horn – Radio microphone

ICU – Intensive-care unit

Intubate – To thread a hollow tube down into the windpipe to facilitate breathing.

IV – Intravenous injection

KIA – Killed in action

LOH – (pronounced loach) Light observation helicopter

LRRP – Long-range reconnaissance patrol. Now called LRP (long-range patrol). Initially four- or five-man teams that would go out for recon; now ten- to twenty-man ambush patrols.

LZ – Landing zone

M-16 – American 5.56-mm infantry rifle

M-60 – American 7.62-machine gun

MACV – Military Assistance Command Vietnam

Med Cap – Medical civil assistance program for Vietnamese civilians

MOS – Military occupational specialty

NCO – Noncommissioned officer

Nephrectomy – Surgical removal of a kidney

NPD – Night perimeter defense

NVA – North Vietnamese Army

OR – Operating room

Point – The lead man on a patrol

RPD – A 7.62-mm Communist machine gun with a 100-round, belt-operated drum that fires the same round as the AK-47.

RPG – A Communist self-propelled rocket.

SF – Special Forces

SI – Seriously ill

Slick – Helicopter for transporting troops

TAC – Tactical air strikes

Thorazine – A tranquilizer

Titers – Amount of anti-body in a serum

TOC – Tactical operation center, usually battalion level and above

Track – Any vehicle that moves on treads instead of wheels

Triage – The sorting out of patients according to the criticalness of their needs, i.e., those who need immediate surgery versus those who need only minimal care.

USARV – United States Army Republic of Vietnam

VC – Viet Cong

Vena Cava – The large vein draining blood back to the heart, the superior vena cava draining the whole upper half of the body, and the interior vena cava draining the lower extremities and trunk.

Ventricular Shunts – Tubes, surgically placed, which drain excessive fluid from the ventricles of the brain.

VSI – Very seriously ill. Army designation for those troopers who may die without immediate and definitive medical care.

WP – White phosphorous

References and
Recommended Reading

Forward

"Iraq and Vietnam", *Foreign Affairs*, Nov./Dec. 2005.

Moore, Lt. General Harold G. and Joseph L. Galloway. *We Were Soldiers Once ... and Young*. New York: Random House, 1992.

Moore, Lt. General Harold G. and Joseph L. Galloway. *We Are Soldiers Still* .... Harper, 2008.

Forty Years of War

Bilmes, Linda. "Soldiers Returning from Iraq and Afghanistan: The Long Term Costs." KSG Faculty Research Working Paper Series, Jan. 2007.

Bilmes, Linda and Joseph Stiglitz. *The Three Trillion Dollar War*. W.W. Norton and Company, Feb. 2008.

Hall, Donald. "Distressed Haiku," *The Painted Bed: Poems*. New York: Houghton Mifflin, 2002.

Meyer, Karl E. "Forty Years in the Sand." *Harper's,* June 2005.

Nusbaumer, Steward. "The Cost of War at Walter Reed." *Intervention Magazine*, Oct. 20, 2005.

Pinsky, Robert. "The Things They Carry." *New York Times*, Nov. 4, 2007.

Tanielian, Terri, ed. and Lisa H. Jaycov, ed. "Invisible Wounds of War: Psychological and Cognitive Injuries, Their Consequences, and Services to Assist Recovery." RAND Corporation's Center for Military Health Policy Research, 2008.

The Late Great 1968 / Welcome to the Army

Glasser, Ronald J. *365 Days*. New York: George Braziller, 1971.

Summers, Harry G. *On Strategy: A Critical Analysis of the Vietnam War*. New York: Dell, 1982.

"Vietnam Ten Years Later." *The New Republic*, Special Issue April 29, 1985.

"War Movies." *Vanity Fair*, March 2008.

Zama / The Wounded

Cleland, Max. *Strong at the Broken Places*. Longstreet Press, 2000.

Glasser, Ronald J. *365 Days*. New York: George Braziller, 1971.

The Medics / Then and Now

Cramer, Eric. "Technology Boosting Survival Rate in Iraq." *Army News Service*, Oct. 31, 2003.

De Tocqueville, Alexis. *Democracy in America*. New York: Signet Classic, 2001.

Gawande, Atul. "Casualties of War: Military Care for the Wounded from Iraq and Afghanistan." *New England Journal of Medicine*, Dec. 9, 2004

"Military Medicine Proceedings." U.S. Naval Institute, April 2006.

"Mobile Army Surgical Hospital (MASH): A Military and Surgical Legacy, The." *Journal of the National Medical Association*, Vol. 97, no. 5. May, 2005.

America's Wars / An Autopsy Report

Browdon, Mark. *Blackhawk Down*. Penguin Books, 1997.

Herbert, Bob. "Dangerous Incompetence." *New York Times*, June 30, 2005.

Galloway, Joseph. "Now is the Time for a Clear-Eyed Look at Where We are in Iraq." *Knight-Ridder Newspapers*, June 1, 2005.

Galloway, Joseph. "Learning Lesson of Vietnam All Over Again." *Knight-Ridder Newspapers*, July 6, 2005.

Galloway, Joseph. "Ia Drang: The Battle That Convinced Ho Chi Minh He Could Win." *Vietnam*, Dec. 2010.

Gavin, James A. *On to Berlin*. New York: Viking Press, 1978.

Kitfield, James. *Prodigal Soldiers: How the Generation of Officers Born of Vietnam Revolutionized the American Style of War*. New York: Simon and Schuster, 1995.

Macgregor, Douglas A. *Breaking the Phalanx*. New York: Praeger, 1997.

Macgregor, Douglas A. *Transformation Under Fire: Revolutionizing How America Fights*. New York: Praeger, 2003.

Rich, Frank. "Forget Armor. All You Need is Love." *New York Times*, Jan. 30, 2005.

Ricks, Thomas E. "Where Does Iraq Stand Among U.S. Wars?" *Washington Post*, May 31, 2004.

Med-evacs and Gunships

"Ambroise Paré." http://www.nndb.com/people /561/000096273

Brown, David. "US Military Medicine Use Old and New Techniques to Save Wounded in Afghanistan." *Washington Post*, Nov. 1, 2010.

Brown, David. "US Strategy for Treating Troops in Afghanistan; Iraq: Keep them Moving." *Washington Post*, Nov. 27, 2010.

Chivers, C.J. "Plunging In to Save Lives in a Bloody War." *New York Times*, June 13, 2010.

Fall, Bernard. *Hell in a Very Small Place*. Lippincott, 1966.

Glasser, Ronald J. *365 Days*. New York: George Braziller, 1971.

Kitfield, James. "Ambulance in the Air." *National Journal*, May 2010.

Street Without Joy. Stackpole, 1964.

"US Military Revamps Combat Medic Training and Care." *The Lancet*, Vol. 361, Feb. 8, 2003.

Teleconferencing / More than Six Degrees of Separation

Brown, David. "Teleconferencing From a War Zone Improves Treatment for Wounded Soldiers." *Washington Post*, Oct. 30, 2010.

Nusbaumer, Steward. "The Cost of War at Walter Reed." *Intervention*, Oct. 20, 2005.

Grady, Denise. "The Wounded: Surviving Multiple Injuries." *New York Times*, January 22, 2006.

Misha, Raja. "Amputation Rate for US Troops Twice that of Past Wars." *Boston Globe*, Dec. 9, 2004.

All the Toms / Iraq 2004

"Battle for Khe Sanh." http://www.en.wikipedia.org

"Battle of Fallujah." http://www.en.wikipedia.org

Foss, Christopher R. *The Encyclopedia of Tanks and Armored Fighting Vehicles.* Los Angeles: Thunder Bay Press, 2002.

Glanz, James and Andrew W. Lehren. "With no Uniforms and Lax Oversight, Contractors Menaced All Sides." *New York Times,* Dec. 24, 2010.

Marlantes, Karl. "Matterhorn." *Atlantic Monthly*, 2010.

"Private Gunmen Fed Turmoil." *New York Times,* Oct. 24, 2010.

Rilkins, Dexter. *The Forever War.* New York: Alfred Knopf, 2008.

Stone, Robert. "On the Ground." *New York Times Book Review,* Sept 14, 2008.

Thompson, Peter. *The Real Insider's Guide to Military Basic Training.* Honesdale, PA: Universal, 2003.

Wright, Evan. *Generation Kill.* Penguin, 2004.

Shell Shock / The Shattering of Minds

Farr, Simon. "Ypres and the Great War." http://www.users.globalnet.com

"Herodotus." http://www.en.wikipedia.org

"Irritable Heart of Soldiers and the Origins of Anglo-American Cardiology, The." *New England Journal of Medicine,* Vol. 348, no. 16, April 17, 2003.

Offley, Ed. "Norman Schwarzkopf Braved Minefields in his Personal and Military Life." *Seattle Post Intelligencer,* Oct. 6, 1992.

Matsakis, Aphrodite. "Vietnam Wives: Facing the Challenge of Life with Veterans Suffering Post-Traumatic Stress." San Francisco: Sidran Press, 1996.

Woolsey, Charles F. *The Irritable Heart of Soldiers.* New York: Ashgate Publishers Ltd., 2002.

The Wars Within

Alvarez, Lizetic. "Wartime Soldier, Conflicted Mom." *New York Times,* Sept. 27, 2009.

"Analysis of V.A. Health Care." V.A. Office of Public Health and Environmental Hazards. March 15, 2005.

"Combating the Stigma of Psychological Injuries. *New York Times*, Dec. 27, 2009.

Dewey, Larry. "War and Redemption: Treatment and Recovery in Combat-related Posttraumatic Stress Disorder." Ashgate Publishing, 2004.

Friedman, Matthew. "Post-Traumatic Stress Disorder in the Military Veteran." Psychiatric Clinics of North America. Vol.17, no. 2, June 1994.

Goode, Erica. "After Combat, Victims of an Inner War." *New York Times*, Aug. 2, 2009.

Herbert, Bob. "Wounds You Can't See." *New York Times,* June 24, 2008.

Hoge, Charles et al. "Combat Duty in Iraq and Afghanistan, Mental Health Problems, and Barriers to Care." *The New England Journal of Medicine,* July 1, 2004.

"Pentagon Report Criticizes Troops Mental Health Care." *Washington Post*, June 16, 2007.

Raskind, Murray. "Reduction of Nightmares and other PTSD Symptoms in Combat Veterans by Prazosin: A Placebo-Controlled Study." *American Journal of Psychiatry,* 160:2, Feb. 2003.

Schenwar, Maya. "PTSD Ignored on Active Duty." http://www.truthout.org

Slack, Charles. "The War Inside." *Proto*, Summer 2010.

"Smoother Path Home, A." *Minneapolis Star and Tribune,* Dec. 22, 2007.

Tanielian, Terri, ed. and Lisa H. Jaycov, ed. "Invisible Wounds of War: Psychological and Cognitive Injuries, Their Consequences, and Services to Assist Recovery." RAND Corporation's Center for Military Health Policy Research, 2008.

"Treatment of Posttraumatic Stress Disorder: An Assessment of the Evidence." Institute of Medicine's Committee on Treatment of Posttraumatic Stress Disorder. National Academic Press, 2008.

"Veteran's Mental Health in the Wake of War." *New England Journal of Medicine*. March 31, 2005.

"What's Behind the Rises in Military Suicides." http://www.AOLnews.com April 9, 2011.

Multiple Deployments / Brains at Risk

"Acute Effects and Recovery Time Following Concussion in Collegiate Football Players." *Journal of the American Medical Association*, Vol. 290, pp. 2556-2563, Nov. 19, 2003.

"Afghanistan: Another Round in the IED Game." http://.www.StratFor. com/print/158145.

Amburn, Brad. "Brain Injuries Lead to War Injuries." *United Press International,* July 23, 2004.

Bissinger, Buzz. "Texas Football and the Price of Paralysis." http://www.time. com

"Congress Questions Military Leaders on Suicides, Traumatic Brain Injuries." http://www.propublica.org

"Ex-team Executive Sounds an Alarm About NFL Head Injuries." *New York Times,* Oct.28, 2009.

Guilmette, Thomas J. and Lauria A. Malia. "Concussive understanding and management among New England High School Coaches." *Brain Injury,* 21(10) pp. 1039-1047, Sept. 2007.

Miller, T. Christian and Daniel Zwerdling. "Brain Injuries Remain Undiagnosed in Thousands of Soldiers." http://www.propublica.org

"Polytrauma amd Blast-related Injuries." VA Queri. Minneapolis, MN, June 2006.

Robert, Richard. "Impact on the Brain." *Scientific American Mind,* Dec. 2008/June 2009.

"Suicides of Soldiers Reach High of Nearly Three Decades." *New York Times,* Jan. 30, 2009.

Walsch, Edward. "Vietnam Groups Critical of Bush's VA Budget." *Washington Post,* March 3, 2004.

Ward, Olivia. "A Growing Toll on Battlefield Brains." http://www.thestar. com/article/240721, June 28, 2007.

Vengrow, Michael Captain MC, U.S. Navy. "Saving Limbs and Lives." *U.S. Naval Institute Proceedings,* Feb. 2007.

The Bleeding Wars

Bumiller, Elisabeth. "The War. A Trillion Can be Cheap." *New York Times,* July 25, 2010.

Galloway, Joseph. "Doomed to Repeat History in Afghanistan." *McClatchy Newspapers,* Feb. 27, 2009.

Galloway, Joseph. "Learning the Lessons of Vietnam all over again." *Knight-Ridder Newspapers,* July 6, 2005.

Galloway, Joseph. "Six Lessons for President Obama." *McClatchy Newspapers*, May 8, 2009.

Graham, Bradley. "Every body Counts." *Washington Post*, Oct. 24, 2003.

Graydon, Carter. "The Forgotten War." *Vanity Fair*, June 20, 2005.

Laird, Melvin. "Wars and Public Opinion." *Foreign Affairs*, Nov./ Dec. 2005.

McMaster, H.R. "Learning From Contemporary Conflicts to Prepare for Future Wars." Foreign Policy Research Institute, Fall 2008.

McMaster, H.R. "When Gadgetry Becomes Strategy." *World Affairs*, Winter 2009.

Rich, Frank. "Forget Armor. All You Need Is Love." *New York Times*, Jan. 30, 2005.

"Science Fiction Army, A." Editorial, *New England Journal of Medicine*, March 31, 2005.

Thomas, Evan. "War of Nerves." *Newsweek*, July 4, 2005.

IEDs / Blasts that Kill and Maim

"Artificial Limbs, Real Help." *Minneapolis Star and Tribune*, March 26, 2005.

Arun, Neil. "Shaped Bombs Magnify Iraq Attacks." BBC News, Oct. 10, 2005.

Cernak, Ibolja. "Blast Injuries: Importance, Basic Mechanisms and Consequences." Johns Hopkins University Applied Physics Laboratory, Biomedicine. Sept. 2007.

Dao, James. "Death Visits a Marine Unit, Once called Lucky." *New York Times*, Aug. 7, 2005.

Depalma, Ralph G. "Blast Injuries." *New England Journal of Medicine*, Vol. 352, no. 13, March 31, 2005.

"DoD opens Amputee Care Center in Texas." *Orthotics and Prosthetics Business News*, March 2005.

Dunham, Will. "Another Iraq War Legacy: Badly-wounded U.S. Troops." *Reuters*, Oct. 23, 2005.

Dwyer, Johnny. "The Wounded." *New York Times Magazine*, March 27, 2005.

Edsall, Thomas B. " VA faces 2.6 billion Shortfall in Medical Care." *Washington Post*. June 29, 2005.

Foote, Shelby. *Red River to Appomattox*. New York: Random House.

Galloway, Joseph. "Army is Broken and in Need of Repair." *Knight-Ridder Newspapers*, Oct. 12, 2005.

Galloway, Joseph. "How to Ruin a Great Army in a Short Time." *Knight-Ridder Newspapers*, Sept. 28, 2003.

Galloway, Joseph. "Now's the Time for a Clear-eyed Look at Where We are in Iraq." *Knight-Ridder Newspapers*, June 1, 2005.

Goodman, Amy. "Veterans Return from Iraq Disabled and Homeless." *Democracy Now*, Dec. 13, 2004.

"Invisible Wounded, The." *Salon*, March 8, 2005.

Little, Bernard S. "Walter Reed Breaks Ground for Amputee Training Center." *Army News Service*, November 22, 2004.

Metz, Rachel. "Embracing the Artificial Limb." *Wired News*. February 18, 2005.

Mishra, Raja. "Amputation Rate for US Troops Twice that of Past Wars." *Boston Globe*, Dec. 9, 2004.

"More Americans Dying from Roadside Bombs in Iraq." http://www.realcities.com, July 10, 2005.

Moss, Michael. "Bloodied Marines Sound Off about Want of Armor and Men." *New York Times*, April 25, 2005.

"Need to Improve Post-traumatic Stress Disorder Services." GAO report. February, 2005.

Nusbaumer, Steward. "The Cost of War at Walter Reed." *Intervention*, Oct. 20, 2005.

Okie, Susan. "Traumatic Brain Injury in the War Zone." *New England Journal of Medicine*, Vol. 352, no. 20, May 19, 2005.

Pace, Eric. "General Westmoreland, who led U.S. in Vietnam, dies." *New York Times*, July 19, 2005.

Preazen, Yochi J. "IED Casualties Up Despite Increased Vigilance." *National Journal*, March 3, 2011.

Summers, Harry G. *On Strategy: A Critical Analyis of the Vietnam War*. New York: Dell, 1982.

Vick, Karl. "The Lasting Wounds of War: Roadside bombs have devastated troops and doctors who treat them." *Washington Post*, April 27, 2004.

Traumatic Brain Injury / PTSD / The Invisible Wounds

Alesander, Andrew L. "Diffusion-Tensor Imaging Implicates Pre Frontal Axonal Injury in Executive Function." Neurotherapeutics Author Manuscript; Available in PMC, July 2008.

"Brain Damage" *NFL Roundup/Associated Press /New York Times Sports*, Dec. 11, 2010.

Chepuri, Neeraj B., M.D. "Diffusion Anisotrophy in the Corpus Callosum." *American Journal of Neuroradiology*, 23, pp. 803-808, May 2002.

Chepuri, Neeraj B., M.D. "Diffusion Tensor Imaging and Its Use in Neurosurgery." *Physician to Physician,* Abbott Northwestern Hospital, Winter 2010.

Cullison, Alan. "On Distant Battlefields, Survival Odds Rise Sharply." *Wall Street Journal*, April 3, 2010.

Dao, James. "Gone a Soldier. One Battalion's wrenching Deployment to Afghanistan." *New York Times*, June 27, 2010.

"Dave Duerson's Shooting Reportedly Ruled a Suicide." *Fan House Newswire,* Feb. 19, 2011.

"Deployment and Use of Mental Health Services Among US Army Wives." *New England Journal of Medicine*, pp. 101-117, Jan. 14, 2010.

Eckolm, Erik. "Surge Seen in Numbers of Homeless Veterans." *New York Times*, Nov. 8, 2007.

Filkins, Dexter. "Lost Soldiers." *New York Times*, March 18, 2010.

Flynn, Ramsy. "After the Big Bang." *Hopkins Medicine*, Fall 2010.

Galloway, Joseph. "Disgusting Treatment for Those Whom We Owe So Much." *McClatchy Newspapers*, Feb. 22, 2007.

Grady, Denise. "The Wounded-Surviving Multiple Injuries." *New York Times*, Jan. 22, 2006.

Homer. *The Odyssey*.

"Invisible Wounds: Fighting Post-Traumatic Stress Disorder." *Proto-Massachusetts General Hospital Magazine*, Summer 2010.

Kors, Joshua. "Disposable Soldiers." *The Nation*, April 26, 2010.

Lombardi, Vincent. "Detection of an Infectious Retrovirus XMRV in the Blood Cells of Patients with Chronic Fatigue Syndrome." *Journal of Science*, Vol. 326, #5952 pp. 585-589, Oct. 2009.

"Mental Illness in Deployed Soldiers" Editorial, British Medical Journal, Vol. 335 p. 571, Sept. 22, 2007.

"NMR in Biomedicine." *NMR BioMed*, 19, pp. 476-483, 2006.

Priest, Dana and Anne Hall. "The War Inside." *Washington Post*, June 17, 2007.

Rubin, Elizabeth. "In one moment, Heroism and Heart Break." *New York Times*, Nov. 14, 2011.

Shapiro, Lynn. "Diffusion Tensor Imaging Finds Brain Damage other Tests Miss." http://www.dotmed.com, Sept. 1, 2009.

Stillman, Sarah. "Drinking, Brawling, Hurting." *Washington Post*, Sept. 2, 2007.

"Thousands of GIs Cope with Brain Damage." *Mass. Press/New York Times. com*, Sept. 10, 2007.

Tuller, David. "Study Links Chronic Fatigue to Virus Class." *New York Times*, Aug. 23, 2010.

All the Jakes / Adrift in Afghanistan

Bacevick, Andrew. *Washington Rules: America's Path to Permanent War*. Henry Holt and Company, 2010.

Dao, James. "The End Game in Afghanistan." *New York Times*, March 27, 2011.

Feifer, Gregory. *The Great Gambler: The Soviet War in Afghanistan*. Harper Collins, 2009.

Filkins, Dexter. "The Taliban is Everywhere. The Soldiers are Not." *New York Times*, Jan. 22, 2009.

Finkel, David. *The Good Soldiers*. Sarah Crichton Books, 2009.

"Great Game, The / Afghanistan" Three plays, Guthrie World Stage Series, Sept. 29-Oct. 17, 2010.

"Last Patrol, The: Getting Right Ugly in Afghanistan." *Atlantic Monthly*, Nov. 1 2010.

Ricks, Tom. "Inside an Afghan battle gone wrong. What happened at Wanat." http://www.ricks.foreignpolicy.com, Jan. 28, 2009.

Stanley, Alessandra. "Situation Report: The Dilemma of Afghanistan." *New York Times* (review), Oct. 13. 2009.

Stanton, Doug. *Horse Soldiers*. Scribner, 2009.

Wright, Evan. *Generation Kill.* Putnam Publishing, 2004.

That Deadly Sense of Privilege

Brunswick, Mark. "It Would Be Minnesota Guards' Largest Mobilization Since WWII." *Minneapolis Star Tribune,* Oct. 10, 2005.

Bunting, Josiah. "Class Warfare." *The American Scholar,* Winter 2005.

Cloud, David. "Part-time Forces on Active Duty Decline Steeply." *New York Times,* July 11, 2005.

De Saxe, Maurice. *Reveries on the Art of War.* (1732) ed. and trans. Brig. General Thomas R. Phillips. New York: Dover Publications, 2007.

Gibbon, Edward. *The Decline and Fall of the Roman Empire.* 1776-1781.

Glubb, Sir John. *The Fate of Empires and Search for Survival.* Edinburgh: William Blackwood And Sons, 1976.

Herbert, Bob. "An Army Ready to Snap." *New York Times,* November 10, 2005.

Krugman, Paul. "Too Few, Yet Too Many." *New York Times,* May 30, 2005.

Noonan, Peggy. "The Defense Secretary Who Let Bin Laden Get Away." *Wall Street Journal,* March 12, 2011.

"Pentagon Proposes Rise in Age Limit for Recruits." *New York Times,* July 22, 2005.

Rich, Frank. "The Vietnamization of Bush's Vacation." *New York Times,* August 28, 2005.

Truscott, Lucian K. "The Not-So-Long-Gray Line." *New York Times,* June 28, 2005.

Witmer, John. *Sisters In Arms: A Father Remembers.* Library Lane Publishing, 2010.

All the Carries and Priscillas

"Amazons." http://www.wikipedia.org

Bumiller, Elisabeth. "For Female Marines, Tea Comes with Bullets." *New York Times,* Oct. 3, 2010.

Holmstedt, Kirsten. *Band of Sisters: American Women at War in Iraq.* Stackpole Books, 2007.

Lumpkin, John L. "First Woman Gets Silver Star Since World War II." *Associated Press,* May 27, 2006.

Solaro, Erin. *Women in the Line of Fire*. Seal Press, 2006.

Bullets of Grief / A Prescription for Prevention

Anderson, Kent. *Sympathy for the Devil*. Bantam Publishing, 2000.

Barns, Frank C. *Cartridges of the World: Military and Commercial-11th Edition*. ed. Stan Skinner. Gun Digest Books, 2006.

Is My Junk All Together?

Brown, David. "Amputation and Genital Injuries Increase Sharply Among Soldiers in Afghanistan." *Washington Post*, March 4, 2011.

"Grievous Wounds Increase in Afghan War." http://www.azstarmet.com

Chronicles / Reduxing Vietnam

Sebestyen, Victor. "Transcripts of Defeat." *New York Times* (Op-Ed), Oct. 28, 2009.

INDEX

concussions, 128–29, 132, 136–37, 154–55

see also brain injuries; mild Traumatic Brain Injuries (mTBIs); post-concussion syndrome; traumatic brain injuries (TBIs)

conferences, medical, 80–81

conscription, 196

see also draft

contractors, 97–98

Corpus Callosum, 163

cowardice, 107

see also fear

Crucible, 88

CT scans, 130, 165, 167–68, 169

Damage Control Surgery, 82–84, 84

Decline and Fall of the Roman Empire (Gibbon), 193

deferments, 13–14, 23–24, 196

dehumanization, 122

dementia, 128, 155–56

Demerol, 72

depression, TBIs and, 135

Desert Storm. see First Persian Gulf War; Iraq War

Dewey, Larry, 113–15, 117, 122, 124, 125

Diagnostic and Statistical Manual of Mental Disorders, 113

Diffuse Axonal Injury (DAI), 166–67

Diffusion Tensor Imaging (DTI), 168–70, 172

disability claims, 170–71

distance medicine. see transcontinental care

Down Range to Iraq and Back, 134

draft, 13, 85, 195–96, 197

Duerson, Dave, 128–29

economic status, draft and, 14

Effexor, 125

Elavil, 126

Emergency Medical Technician (EMT) test/training, 69, 75

evacuations. see medical evacuation

executions, for cowardice, 107

Explaining Brain Injury, Blast Injury and PTSD to Children and Teens, 134

extensions of service, 24–27

eye injury, 99–100

"Factor 8," 72

Fallujah, Battles of, 90–95, 219–20

fear, 103–7 passim

Feynman, Richard, 162

First Persian Gulf War
    McMaster on, 141
    medical evacuations and, 68
    PTSD and, 118
    success of, 197
    women in, 213

First World War. see World War I

flashbacks, 50

"the Fog of War," 74, 123

football players, 128–29, 132, 155–56

Foreign Legion, 194

Fort Knox, 88

Fort Rucker, 59

Fort Sam Houston, 15, 16–17, 19

Forward Operating Base Geronimo, 183–84, 185

265